Joint-Preserving Surgery of Ankle Osteoarthritis

Editor

VICTOR VALDERRABANO

FOOT AND ANKLE CLINICS

www.foot.theclinics.com

Consulting Editor
MARK S. MYERSON

September 2013 • Volume 18 • Number 3

ELSEVIER

1600 John F. Kennedy Boulevard • Suite 1800 • Philadelphia, Pennsylvania, 19103-2899

http://www.theclinics.com

FOOT AND ANKLE CLINICS Volume 18, Number 3
September 2013 ISSN 1083-7515, ISBN-13: 978-0-323-18854-8

Editor: Jennifer Flynn-Briggs

Foot and Ankle Clinics (ISSN 1083-7515) is published quarterly by Elsevier, Inc., 360 Park Avenue South, New York, NY 10010-1710. Months of issue are March, June, September, and December. Periodicals postage paid at New York, NY, and additional mailing offices. Subscription price per year is $299.00 (US individuals), $401.00 (US institutions), $148.00 (US students), $341.00 (Canadian individuals), $473.00 (Canadian institutions), $204.00 (Canadian students), $439.00 (foreign individuals), $473.00 (foreign institutions), and $204.00 (foreign students). To receive student/resident rate, orders must be accompanied by name of affiliated institution, date of term, and the *signature* of program/residency coordinator on institution letterhead. Orders will be billed at individual rate until proof of status is received. Foreign air speed delivery is included in all *Clinics* subscription prices. All prices are subject to change without notice. **POSTMASTER:** Send address changes to *Foot and Ankle Clinics*, Elsevier Health Sciences Division, Subscription Customer Service, 3251 Riverport Lane, Maryland Heights, MO 63043. **Customer Service: 1-800-654-2452 (US and Canada). From outside of the United States and Canada, call 314-447-8871. Fax: 314-447-8029. E-mail: JournalsCustomerService-usa@ elsevier.com (for print support); JournalsOnlineSupport-usa@elsevier.com (for online support).**

Reprints. For copies of 100 or more, of articles in this publication, please contact the Commercial Reprints Department, Elsevier Inc., 360 Park Avenue South, New York, NY 10010-1710. Tel.: 212-633-3874; Fax: 212-633-3820; E-mail: reprints@elsevier.com.

Printed and bound by CPI Group (UK) Ltd, Croydon, CR0 4YY

Transferred to digital print 2013

Contributors

CONSULTING EDITOR

MARK S. MYERSON, MD
Director, The Institute for Foot and Ankle Reconstruction, Mercy Medical Center, Baltimore, Maryland

EDITOR

VICTOR VALDERRABANO, MD, PhD
Professor and Chairman, Orthopaedic Department, Osteoarthritis Research Center Basel, University Hospital of Basel, University of Basel, Basel, Switzerland

AUTHORS

ANNUNZIATO AMENDOLA, MD
Kim and John Callaghan Endowed Professor, Director of Sports Medicine Center, Department of Orthopaedics and Rehabilitation, University of Iowa Hospitals and Clinics, Iowa City, Iowa

ALEXEJ BARG, MD
Attending Surgeon, Orthopaedic Department, Osteoarthritis Research Center Basel, University Hospital of Basel, University of Basel, Basel, Switzerland; Research Fellow, Department of Orthopaedics, Harold K. Dunn Orthopaedic Research Laboratory, University Orthopaedic Center, University of Utah, Salt Lake City, Utah

DOUGLAS N. BEAMAN, MD
Orthopaedic Surgeon, Summin Orthopaedics LLP, Portland, Oregon

DAVID M. DARE, MD
Resident Physician, Department of Orthopaedic Surgery, Hospital for Special Surgery, New York, New York

JONATHAN T. DELAND, MD
Attending Orthopaedic Surgeon, Division of Foot and Ankle Surgery, Hospital for Special Surgery; Professor of Clinical Orthopaedic Surgery, Department of Orthopaedic Surgery, Weill Cornell Medical College, New York, New York

A. LEE DELLON, MD, PhD
Professor of Plastic Surgery and Neurosurgery, Johns Hopkins University, Baltimore; Dellon Institutes for Peripheral Nerve Surgery, Towson, Maryland

NORMAN ESPINOSA, MD
Head of Foot and Ankle Surgery, Department of Orthopaedics, Balgrist Hospital, University of Zurich, Zurich, Switzerland

ILARIO FULCO, MD
Plastic, Reconstructive and Aesthetic Surgery, Hand Surgery, University Hospital, Basel, Switzerland

MARCEL GLOYER, MD
Resident, Orthopaedic Department, University Hospital of Basel, University of Basel, Basel, Switzerland

ANDREAS GOHRITZ, MD
Plastic, Reconstructive and Aesthetic Surgery, Hand Surgery, University Hospital, Basel, Switzerland

HEATH B. HENNINGER, PhD
Assistant Professor, Department of Orthopaedics, Harold K. Dunn Orthopaedic Research Laboratory, University Orthopaedic Center, University of Utah, Salt Lake City, Utah

BEAT HINTERMANN, MD
Associated Professor and Director, Orthopaedic Department, Clinic of Orthopaedic Surgery and Traumatology, Kantonsspital Baselland, Liestal, Switzerland

MACALUS V. HOGAN, MD
Assistant Professor of Orthopaedic Surgery, Division of Foot and Ankle Surgery, Department of Orthopaedic Surgery, University of Pittsburgh Medical Center, Pittsburgh, Pennsylvania

THOMAS HÜGLE, MD, PhD
Assistant Professor, Orthopaedic Department, Osteoarthritis Research Center Basel, University Hospital of Basel, University of Basel, Basel, Switzerland

DANIEL KALBERMATTEN, MD, PhD
Plastic, Reconstructive and Aesthetic Surgery, Hand Surgery, University Hospital, Basel, Switzerland

MARKUS KNUPP, MD
Assistant Professor and Senior Attending Surgeon, Clinic of Orthopaedic Surgery, Kantonsspital Baselland, Liestal, Switzerland

FABIAN G. KRAUSE, MD
Department of Orthopaedic Surgery, Inselspital, University of Berne, Freiburgstrasse, Berne, Switzerland

HORISBERGER MONIKA, MD
Attending Surgeon, Orthopaedic Department, University Hospital of Basel, University of Basel, Basel, Switzerland

MARK S. MYERSON, MD
Director, Institute for Foot and Ankle Reconstruction, Mercy Medical Center, Baltimore, Maryland

CORINA NÜESCH, PhD
Osteoarthritis Research Center, University Hospital of Basel, University of Basel, Basel, Switzerland

GEERT I. PAGENSTERT, MD
Senior Attending Surgeon and Assistant Professor, Orthopaedic Department, University Hospital of Basel, University of Basel, Basel, Switzerland

JOCHEN PAUL, MD
Attending Surgeon, Orthopaedic Department, University Hospital of Basel, University of Basel, Basel, Switzerland

PHINIT PHISITKUL, MD
Department of Orthopaedics and Rehabilitation, University of Iowa Hospitals and Clinics, Iowa City, Iowa

STEVEN M. RAIKIN, MD
Director, Foot and Ankle Service, Professor of Orthopaedic Surgery, Department of Orthopaedic Surgery, Rothman Institute of Orthopedics, Thomas Jefferson University Hospital, Philadelphia, Pennsylvania

CHARLES L. SALTZMAN, MD
Louis S. Perry Endowed Presidential Professor and Chairman, University Orthopaedic Center, University of Utah, Salt Lake City, Utah

DIRK J. SCHAEFER, MD, PhD
Plastic, Reconstructive and Aesthetic Surgery, Hand Surgery, University Hospital, Basel, Switzerland

TIMO SCHMID, MD
Department of Orthopaedic Surgery, Inselspital, University of Berne, Freiburgstrasse, Berne, Switzerland

JOSHUA N. TENNANT, MD, MPH
Department of Orthopaedics and Rehabilitation, University of Iowa Hospitals and Clinics, Iowa City, Iowa

MATHIAS TREMP, MD
Plastic, Reconstructive and Aesthetic Surgery, Hand Surgery, University Hospital, Basel, Switzerland

VICTOR VALDERRABANO, MD, PhD
Professor and Chairman, Orthopaedic Department, Osteoarthritis Research Center Basel, University Hospital of Basel, University of Basel, Basel, Switzerland

MARTIN WIEWIORSKI, MD
Resident, Orthopaedic Department, University Hospital of Basel, University of Basel, Basel, Switzerland; Research Fellow, Center for Advanced Orthopaedic Studies, Beth Israel Deaconess Medical Center, Harvard Medical School, Boston, Massachusetts

BRIAN S. WINTERS, MD
Fellow in Foot and Ankle Surgery, Department of Orthopaedic Surgery, Rothman Institute of Orthopaedics, Thomas Jefferson University Hospital, Philadelphia, Pennsylvania

JACOB R. ZIDE, MD
Institute for Foot and Ankle Reconstruction, Mercy Medical Center, Baltimore, Maryland

Contents

symptoms. Discussion includes the role of diagnostic arthroscopy and adjunctive use of arthroscopy with other modalities. The section on the authors' preferred technique describes our current operative and perioperative strategies in detail.

For select patients, distraction ankle arthroplasty may be a promising treatment approach for ankle osteoarthritis; however, there is still limited literature addressing its efficacy and clinical long-term results. In this article, the literature regarding the outcome after ankle distraction arthroscopy is reviewed, the indications and contraindication for this procedure are listed, our surgical technique is described, and our preliminary results with this procedure are presented.

The goal of osteotomy in the treatment of varus ankle arthritis is to shift the forces imparted to the ankle to a portion of the joint that is not involved in the degenerative process. The redistribution of loads and stresses seen by the tibiotalar joint can be approached either above or below the ankle with an osteotomy of the tibia or calcaneus. Evaluation of the deformity as being subtalar, supramalleolar, or a combination allows the surgeon to best address the increased joint stresses, thereby reducing the risk of failure of the osteotomy.

Patients with posttraumatic ankle osteoarthritis (OA) typically present with asymmetric involvement of the tibiotalar joint, resulting in valgus or varus deformity of the ankle and hindfoot. Without appropriate treatment, patients with asymmetric ankle OA typically develop full end-stage ankle OA. Ankles with valgus deformities suffer from a lateral joint overload with subsequent lateral tibiotalar joint degeneration, which causes further lateral load shift. In these cases, patients may benefit from joint-preserving realignment surgery to unload the degenerated lateral area and normalize joint biomechanics. This article describes the authors' algorithm for the treatment of patients with asymmetric valgus ankle OA.

A varus or valgus talar tilt that increases under weight-bearing is commonly seen in osteoarthritic ankles. Loss of peritalar stability may be the underlying cause for the talus shifting and rotating on the calcaneonavicular surfaces, as given by applied forces. The instability pattern and the resulting deformity can be assessed and classified using weight-bearing conventional radiographs. Appropriate osseous balancing may be the most appropriate treatment to restore a regular position of talus within the ankle mortise. In cases with severe peritalar instability, subtalar fusion may be advised. Soft tissue reconstruction may be needed to achieve physiologic balance of the hindfoot complex.

Varus and valgus ankle deformities represent a challenge to the foot and ankle surgeons. The presence of degenerative changes of the tibiotalar joint articular surfaces introduces an additional layer of complexity. Reconstruction of such deformities requires a customized approach to each patient. Surgical intervention often requires joint-sparing realignment, arthroplasty, and/or arthrodesis, depending on the severity of deformity and the joint surface integrity. The ligamentous stability of the ankle plays an essential role in the preservation and optimization of function. This article reviews the role of deltoid and lateral ligament reconstruction in the treatment of varus and valgus ankle osteoarthritis.

The surgical management of young patients with large osteochondral lesions of the talus or end-stage osteoarthritis of the ankle joint presents a challenge to the orthopedic surgeon because these are well-recognized sources of pain and dysfunction. Procedures designed to address these disorders either have a limited role because of poor success rates or have significant implications, such as with the total ankle arthroplasty. Fresh osteochondral allografts allow defective tissue to be anatomically matched and reconstructed through transplantation. This article presents an overview of fresh osteochondral allografts, as well as potential concerns with their use, and summarizes the current literature.

Local cartilage or osteochondral degeneration of the ankle are common, painful posttraumatic conditions in young, sport-active patients. Conservative treatment of the acute initial stage of local cartilage or osteochondral damage might be indicated, but commonly fails in the presence of local or asymmetric osteoarthritic disease. Many surgical treatment methods are available for the orthopedic surgeon, which show satisfactory short-term to mid-term results. However, the scientific evidence for these procedures is weak. This article discusses the commonly used methods for cartilage and osteochondral repair and new upcoming methods, plus the role of concomitant disorders of the ankle joint.

This article discusses the lack of scientific evidence regarding the treatment of failed joint-preserving surgery. Most of the concepts of treatment derive from treatment modalities in trauma and orthopedic surgery. The main question for the foot and ankle specialist is whether the joint can be salvaged. The definition of failure is difficult. Therefore pain reported by the patient is the main symptom that dictates the course of treatment. Whenever possible the joint should be maintained. However, if pain is associated with global radiographic osteoarthritis, total ankle replacement or fusions are the only means to solve the problem.

FOOT AND ANKLE CLINICS

Preface

Joint-Preserving Surgery of Ankle Osteoarthritis

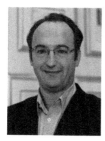

Victor Valderrabano, MD, PhD
Editor

In the last decades, substantial advances in understanding the ankle joint anatomy and biomechanics as well as the pathogenesis of ankle osteoarthritis (OA) have led to new approaches in the treatment of ankle OA. While joint-wide end-stage ankle OA is typically treated by total ankle arthroplasty or ankle arthrodesis (ie, joint-sacrificing surgeries), asymmetric degenerative ankle OA can be treated by joint-preserving surgery (ie, by osteotomies together with possible osteochondral repair, ligament and tendon reconstructions, and others).

Joint-preserving ankle surgery has an exceptional position in the treatment algorithm of ankle OA. In many cases, it may decelerate or even stop the further development of the degenerative arthritic process. This means, in turn, that mid- or long-term postponing of total ankle arthroplasty or ankle arthrodesis is possible. Therefore, it has been a pleasure and a big honor, but also a great motivation, for me to participate as guest editor of this issue of *Foot and Ankle Clinics of North America* highlighting different joint-preserving procedures in patients with degenerative changes of the ankle joint.

The choice of an appropriate treatment algorithm and correct indication in patients with beginning, mid-stage, asymmetric ankle OA is not simple and requires the accordant experience in foot and ankle surgery. Furthermore, the complex underlying biomechanics of concomitant deformities in patients with asymmetric ankle OA needs to be recognized and properly analyzed to be able to plan the surgical procedure step by step. In most cases, there is no "cookbook" solution of the underlying problem—each case should be analyzed and assessed individually. The underlying osseous deformity should be assessed and quantified clinically and radiographically. The origin of the deformity needs to be recognized and addressed properly. Furthermore, all concomitant problems including degenerative changes of the neighboring joints and ligamental instability have to be addressed to ensure success of the surgical procedure and good and satisfied functional results.

Foot Ankle Clin N Am 18 (2013) xiii–xiv
http://dx.doi.org/10.1016/j.fcl.2013.06.013
1083-7515/13/$ – see front matter © 2013 Published by Elsevier Inc.

foot.theclinics.com

While total ankle arthroplasty and ankle arthrodesis are well-established surgical procedures, the realignment osteotomy around the ankle joint is a relatively new procedure. Professor Takakura was one of the first orthopedic surgeons to present his experience with supramalleolar osteotomies in the British volume of *Journal of Bone and Joint Surgery* in the year 1995. The promising postoperative results encouraged other working groups to use this surgical technique as possible treatment options in patients with asymmetric ankle OA.

Due to the outstanding contributions of all the authors and coauthors, this issue includes excellent clinical and scientific review articles addressing diverse facets of joint-preserving ankle surgery and different surgical techniques in patients with beginning or mid-stage ankle OA. The issue starts with basic subjects: etiology and diagnostics of ankle OA, including physical examination and different imaging modalities (Barg et al) followed by the review addressing the biomechanics of asymmetric ankle OA and its joint-preserving surgery (Nueesch et al). In most cases, the treatment protocol starts with conservative nonoperative measures, including physiotherapy, as it has been shown in the review by Krause et al. In patients with beginning ankle OA and painful ankle impingement especially, the arthroscopic debridement may provide substantial pain relief and satisfied functional results (Amendola et al). Another therapeutic option in patients with relatively congruent tibiotalar joint and preserved ankle joint mobility is the distraction ankle arthroplasty (Barg and Saltzman). A step-by-step surgical treatment algorithm in patients with varus and valgus ankle OA has been highlighted in reviews by Myerson et al and Valderrabano et al, respectively. The complexity of the etiology in patients with peritalar instability has been described in the review by Hintermann et al. Deland et al reviewed the high clinical importance of the concomitant ligamental problems. Raikin et al shared their experience of the use of allograft in this patient cohort. Wiewiorski et al performed a thorough review highlighting the different osteochondral reconstruction procedures. Finally, two last reviews of this issue (Espinosa et al and Schaefer et al) describe how to deal with the patients where joint-preserving surgery failed and did not lead to expected postoperative pain relief and functional improvement.

Finally, I would like to thank and congratulate all my colleagues participating in this project, resulting in a high-quality issue highlighting different important aspects of joint-preserving ankle surgery. Furthermore, I would like to thank Mark Myerson, for his kind invitation to serve as guest editor of this issue, and the staff of Elsevier for excellent assistance in preparing and accomplishing this work-intensive project. I hope this issue will find interest in the foot-and-ankle-surgeon community.

Victor Valderrabano, MD, PhD
Orthopaedic Department
and Osteoarthritis Research Center Basel
University Hospital of Basel
University of Basel
Spialstrasse 21
4031 Basel, Switzerland

E-mail address:
victor.valderrabano@usb.ch

Ankle Osteoarthritis
Etiology, Diagnostics, and Classification

Alexej Barg, MD[a,b,]*, Geert I. Pagenstert, MD[c],
Thomas Hügle, MD, PhD[a], Marcel Gloyer, MD[c],
Martin Wiewiorski, MD[c,d], Heath B. Henninger, PhD[b],
Victor Valderrabano, MD, PhD[a,]*

KEYWORDS

- Ankle osteoarthritis • Etiology of ankle osteoarthritis
- Posttraumatic ankle osteoarthritis • Classification of ankle osteoarthritis
- Diagnostics of ankle osteoarthritis

KEY POINTS

- Osteoarthritis is a constantly growing problem in health care with approximately 1% of the world's adult population affected by ankle osteoarthritis.
- Previous trauma is the most common reason for ankle osteoarthritis.
- The mental and physical disability associated with end-stage ankle osteoarthritis is at least as severe as that associated with end-stage osteoarthritis of the hip joint.
- Conventional radiological imaging of ankle osteoarthritis include 4 weight-bearing radiographs: anteroposterior and lateral views of the foot, mortise view of the ankle, and Saltzman view of the hindfoot.
- Single-photon emission computed tomography/computed tomography (SPECT-CT) may help to evaluate the extend of degenerative changes of the foot/ankle joints and their biological activities.
- The most common current ankle osteoarthritis classification systems are based on radiographic evaluation of degenerative changes of the tibiotalar joint.

The authors have nothing to disclose.
[a] Orthopaedic Department, Osteoarthritis Research Center Basel, University Hospital of Basel, University of Basel, Spitalstrasse 21, Basel CH-4031, Switzerland; [b] Harold K. Dunn Orthopaedic Research Laboratory, University Orthopaedic Center, University of Utah, 590 Wakara Way, Salt Lake City, UT 84108, USA; [c] Orthopaedic Department, University Hospital of Basel, University of Basel, Spitalstrasse 21, Basel CH-4031, Switzerland; [d] Center for Advanced Orthopaedic Studies, Beth Israel Deaconess Medical Center, Harvard Medical School, 330 Brookline Avenue, RN 115, Boston, MA 02215, USA
* Corresponding authors. Orthopaedic Department, Osteoarthritis Research Center Basel, University Hospital of Basel, University of Basel, Spitalstrasse 21, Basel CH-4031, Switzerland.
E-mail addresses: victor.valderrabano@usb.ch; alexej.barg@usb.ch

Foot Ankle Clin N Am 18 (2013) 411–426
http://dx.doi.org/10.1016/j.fcl.2013.06.001
1083-7515/13/$ – see front matter © 2013 Elsevier Inc. All rights reserved.

foot.theclinics.com

ETIOLOGY OF ANKLE OSTEOARTHRITIS

Osteoarthritis (OA) as a debilitating chronic disease is a growing problem in health care.[1–3] Approximately 1% of the world's adult population is affected by ankle OA, which results in pain, dysfunction, and impaired mobility.[4,5] The mental and physical disability associated with end-stage ankle OA is at least as severe as that associated with end-stage hip OA.[4] Whereas the etiology of hip and knee OA is well understood and highlighted in numerous clinical studies, research related to ankle OA is limited.[5] The knowledge and analysis of the underlying etiology are important for selecting the best treatment strategy and are keys to achieving satisfactory long-term results and avoiding postoperative complications.

Unlike the hip and knee, the ankle joint is rarely affected by primary OA. Instead, numerous clinical and epidemiologic studies have identified previous trauma as the most common origin of ankle OA. Patients with posttraumatic OA are generally younger than patients with primary OA (**Fig. 1**).[5–9] An epidemiologic study of patients presenting with disabling hip, knee, and ankle OA showed that 1.6% of patients with hip OA, 9.8% of patients with knee OA, and 79.5% of patients with ankle OA had a verified history of 1 or more joint injuries.[10] Saltzman and colleagues[6] evaluated 639 patients presenting with painful end-stage ankle OA (Kellgren grade 3 or 4). In this cohort, 445 patients (70%) had posttraumatic OA, 76 (12%) had rheumatoid OA, and 46 (7%) had primary ankle OA. While rotational ankle fractures were identified as the most common reason for posttraumatic ankle OA (164 patients), previous ligamental injuries were also found to be a cause of ankle OA in 126 patients.[6] Repetitive ankle sprains in sports (eg, soccer) are the main cause of ligamentous posttraumatic ankle OA with concomitant varus hindfoot deformity.[11] These trends were confirmed by Valderrabano and colleagues,[5] who evaluated the etiology of ankle OA in 390 consecutive patients (406 ankles) with painful end-stage ankle OA. Most patients (78%) presented with posttraumatic OA. In this study, malleolar fractures were the most common reason for degenerative changes in ankle joint (157 patients), followed by ankle ligament lesions (ligamentous posttraumatic ankle OA; 60 patients). Only 31 patients were affected by primary OA, whereas secondary OA was seen as the more common cause of end-stage ankle OA (46 patients).[5] Secondary OA has also been associated with a variety of underlying diseases or disorders, such as rheumatoid disease, hemochromatosis, hemophilia, gout, neuropathic diseases, avascular talus necrosis, osteochondral lesions, and postinfectious arthritis (**Table 1**).[5,6] In all 3 main etiology groups the obesity was identified as a risk factor for OA development, as was shown in an epidemiologic study including 1411 adults.[12]

Results of the literature review are summarized in **Table 2**, which shows causes of ankle OA as an indication for realignment surgery in patients with asymmetric ankle OA.

EARLY ONSET AND DEVELOPMENT OF POSTTRAUMATIC ANKLE OSTEOARTHRITIS

The etiology of posttraumatic OA and its pathomechanical basics have been studied extensively. Posttraumatic OA may result from irreversible cartilage damage that occurred at the time of injury, and chronic cartilage overloading resulting from articular incongruity and instability.[21,22] Horisberger and colleagues[23] identified the latency time between injury and end-stage posttraumatic ankle OA as 20.9 years, with a range between 1 and 52 years, in a clinical study including 257 patients (270 ankles) with painful end-stage ankle OA. The major factors influencing the observed latency time were the type of fracture, complications arising in the healing phase, age at the time of injury, and a varus malalignment of the hindfoot.[23] Lübbeke and colleagues[24] conducted a retrospective cohort study including 372 consecutive patients treated by

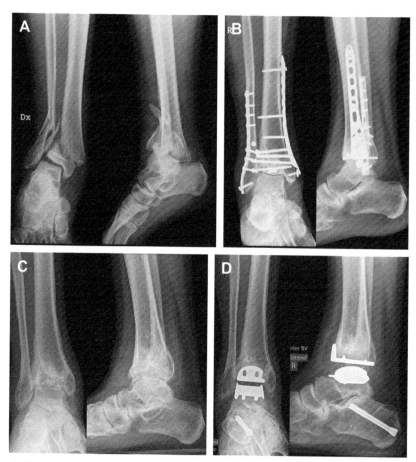

Fig. 1. Posttraumatic ankle osteoarthritis. (*A*) Anteroposterior and lateral radiographs of a 24-year-old male patient with displaced lower leg fracture sustained from a fall down stairs. (*B*) Weight-bearing radiographs show complete fracture healing after open reduction and internal fixation 10 months postoperatively. (*C*) Hardware removal was performed 23 months postoperatively. Despite the anatomic reduction and uneventful healing of the fracture, significant degenerative changes of the tibiotalar joint are visible. (*D*) All attempts at conservative treatment were unsuccessful, therefore 32 months after the accident the total ankle replacement using HINTEGRA was performed. (*From* Barg A, Knupp M, Henninger HB, et al. Total ankle replacement using HINTEGRA, an unconstrained, three-component system: surgical technique and pitfalls. Foot Ankle Clin 2012;17(4):608; with permission.)

open reduction and internal fixation for malleolar fracture. In more than one-third of all patients advanced radiographic ankle OA was observed, especially following Weber C fractures and associated medial malleolar fractures. The latency time between injury and ankle OA ranged between 12 and 22 years. Further identified risk factors for OA development were substantial fracture dislocation, increasing body mass index, age 30 years or older, length of time since surgery.[24] Stufkens and colleagues[25] performed a long-term follow-up study of a consecutive, prospective cohort of 288 ankle fractures. The initial cartilage damage seen arthroscopically following an ankle fracture was identified as an independent predictor of the development of ankle OA.[25]

Table 1
Causes of secondary osteoarthritis

Cause of Secondary Osteoarthritis	Presumed Mechanism of Osteoarthritis Development
Joint injuries	Damage to articular surface and/or residual joint incongruity and instability
Joint dysplasias (developmental and hereditary joint and cartilage dysplasias)	Abnormal joint shape and/or abnormal articular cartilage
Aseptic necrosis	Bone necrosis leads to collapse of the articular surface, resulting in joint incongruity
Rheumatoid arthritis	Autoimmune disease, destruction of articular cartilage
Acromegaly	Overgrowth of articular cartilage resulting in joint incongruity and/or abnormal cartilage
Paget disease	Distortion and incongruity of joints caused by bone remodeling
Ehlers-Danlos syndrome	Joint instability
Gaucher disease (hereditary deficiency of the enzyme glucocerebrosidase leading to accumulation of glucocerebroside)	Bone necrosis or pathologic bone fracture leading to joint incongruity
Stickler syndrome (progressive hereditary arthro-ophthalmopathy)	Abnormal joint and/or articular cartilage development
Joint infection (inflammation)	Complete or partial destruction of articular cartilage
Hemophilia	Multiple repetitive joint hemorrhages
Hemochromatosis (excess iron deposition in multiple tissues)	Mechanism unknown
Gout, calcium pyrophosphate deposition disease	Accumulation of calcium pyrophosphate crystals in articular cartilage
Ochronosis (hereditary deficiency of enzyme, homogentisic acid oxidase leading to accumulation of homogentisic acid)	Deposition of homogentisic acid polymers in articular cartilage
Neuropathic arthropathy (Charcot joints: syphilis, diabetes mellitus, syringomyelia, meningomyelocele, leprosy, congenital insensitivity to pain, amyloidosis)	Loss of proprioception and joint sensation results in increased impact loading and torsion, joint instability, and intra-articular fractures

Data from Buckwalter JA, Martin JA. Osteoarthritis. Adv Drug Deliv Rev 2006;58(2):153; and Buckwalter JA, Mankin HJ. Articular cartilage: degeneration and osteoarthritis, repair, regeneration, and transplantation. Instr Course Lect 1998;47:489.

McKinley and colleagues[22] have shown in a cadaver model that a step-off incongruity of the anterolateral distal tibia leads to substantial increases in contact stresses, contact-stress directional gradients, and contact-stress rates of change. In another study, the same group showed that instability in the presence of joint incongruity dramatically increased the transient contact-stress directional gradients when compared with cadaver specimens with incongruity alone.[26] Similar findings were observed in the study by Tochigi and colleagues,[27] who have shown that even very small instability events, some of which may not be detectable clinically or as a kinematic abnormality, may substantially lead to aberration of dynamic contact stresses.[27] Anderson and colleagues[28] performed a clinical study including 10 ankles treated for

Table 2
Etiology of ankle osteoarthritis as indication for realignment surgery in patients with asymmetric ankle osteoarthritis

Authors,[Ref.] Year	Patients	Procedure
Cheng et al,[13] 2001	Primary (12) and posttraumatic (6) OA with varus deformity	Supramalleolar media opening-wedge osteotomy with fibular osteotomy (18)
Lee et al,[14] 2011	Primary (8) and posttraumatic (ligamentous) (8) OA with varus deformity	Supramalleolar medial opening-wedge osteotomy with fibular osteotomy (16)
Harstall et al,[15] 2007	Posttraumatic (8) and secondary (1) OA with varus deformity	Supramalleolar lateral closing-wedge osteotomy (9)
Neumann et al,[16] 2007	Primary (18), posttraumatic (7), and secondary OA due to clubfoot deformity with varus deformity (2)	Supramalleolar lateral closing-wedge osteotomy (27)
Pagenstert et al,[17] 2007	Posttraumatic (35) OA with varus (13) or valgus (22) deformity	Supramalleolar osteotomy (35)
Pagenstert et al,[18] 2009	Posttraumatic (22) OA with valgus deformity	Supramalleolar medial closing-wedge osteotomy (22)
Takakura et al,[19] 1995	Primary (idiopathic) OA with varus deformity (18)	Supramalleolar medial opening-wedge osteotomy (18)
Takakura et al,[20] 1998	Posttraumatic varus deformity (9)	Supramalleolar medial opening-wedge osteotomy (9)

tibial plafond fracture. The investigators identified the incongruous reduction of intra-articular fracture as an important risk factor for the development of posttraumatic ankle OA.[28]

Tochigi and colleagues[29] used 7 normal human ankles harvested immediately following amputation. All specimens were subjected to a transarticular compressive impaction mimicking the injury mechanism typically observed in tibial plafond fractures. Immediately postfracture, chondrocyte death in the superficial layers was the highest in fracture-edge regions. The progression of cell death over the next 48 hours was also significantly higher in fracture-edge regions than in nonfracture regions of the ankle-joint surface.[29]

There is no doubt that not only the inaccurate reduction of intra-articular fractures but also the osteochondral impact at the injury moment results in progressive post-traumatic OA.[30] The onset and development of posttraumatic ankle OA has been the subject of intensive biomechanical and morphologic research identifying incongruity and instability as the most important risk factors for this pathologic entity. In the ankle joint as a weight-bearing joint, osteoarthritic process and biomechanics are strongly linked: altered loading patterns, increased intra-articular and periarticular mechanical forces, and changed biomechanics are substantial contributing factors in the initiation and progression of ankle OA.[31]

DIAGNOSTICS OF ANKLE OSTEOARTHRITIS
Clinical Study of Ankle Osteoarthritis

The functional limitations in patients with ankle OA are often substantial and should not be trivialized. Glazebrook and colleagues[4] performed a Level I study comparing the health-related quality of life between patients with end-stage ankle and hip OA.

Patients with ankle OA had significantly worse mental component summary scores, role-physical scores, and general health score, as assessed using Short Form-36 (SF-36) generic outcome instruments. The investigators concluded that the mental and physical disability associated with end-stage ankle OA should not be underestimated, as it is at least as severe as that associated with end-stage OA of the hip joint.[4]

Another study confirmed substantial functional impairments in patients with end-stage ankle OA.[32] Patients with end-stage degenerative changes of the tibiotalar joint had significantly reduced ankle range of motion and impaired gait parameters. These findings were consistent with the previous literature.[33–35] The overall physical function, as assessed using the SF-36 score (Physical Function), was also substantially impaired, which may partially explain the reduced public walking and sustained higher-intensity walking with reduced self-perceived function in this cohort.[32]

Most patients with ankle OA seek medical help because of progressive joint pain. Patients often describe the pain as a deep aching within the tibiotalar joint. The pain may be localized (eg, anterolateral) or general, with pain around the whole hindfoot complex. All patients can be divided into 2 main groups: those with slowly and rapidly progressive ankle OA.

The pain may have a different time-related character and may depend on the bearing of the ankle joint. Therefore, the authors suggest use of a visual analog scale (VAS)[36] to address different aspects of pain level: overall pain, starting pain, stress pain, resting pain, and pain at night.[37,38] Some patients describe themselves as "weathermen," as the pain may increase with changes in the weather. Pains associated with daily or sporting activities may typically begin immediately or shortly after the beginning of joint use, and may persist for hours or even days after cessation of activities.[1] In patients with early degenerative changes of the tibiotalar joint, the pain usually persists during the day at higher loading. However, in the more advanced stages of OA the pain may also occur at rest and during the night, and may awaken patients from sleep.

The routine physical examination includes careful inspection of the entire hindfoot complex and foot. Ankle alignment should be assessed clinically with the patient standing.[39,40] Frigg and colleagues[41] has demonstrated that the visual judgment is inadequate to determine the hindfoot alignment because it predicts the radiographic alignment in less than half of clinical cases. Substantial muscle atrophy of the lower leg may occur in patients with midstage and end-stage ankle OA, as has been shown by Valderrabano and colleagues[35,42,43]

One of the first clinical signs of ankle OA includes stiffness or a substantial decrease of overall range of motion of the tibiotalar joint. The authors determine ankle range of motion using a goniometer placed along the lateral border of the leg and foot.[44,45] All goniometer measurements are performed in the weight-bearing position, comparable with the method described by Lindsjö and colleagues.[46] The accuracy of the goniometric measurements has been assessed by direct comparison with ankle range-of-motion measurements obtained from radiographs.[44,45,47,48] Reduced ankle range of motion may have different causes including incongruity or loss of articular cartilage, contractures of periarticular ligaments and capsular structures, muscle spasm and contracture, and osteophytes or intra-articular fragments (loose bodies) of cartilage.[1] Patients with progressive ankle OA may also present with crepitus, joint effusions, and joint tenderness. Osteophytes can cause palpable tenderness, especially on the anteromedial and anteromedial aspects of the ankle joint. The authors assess the hindfoot stability manually, with the patient sitting, using standard talar tilt and anterior drawer test.[49]

Radiological Imaging of Ankle Osteoarthritis

The authors routinely perform a 4 film series of conventional radiographs including anteroposterior and lateral views of the foot, mortise view of the ankle, and Saltzman view[50] of the hindfoot (**Fig. 2**). Only weight-bearing radiographs of the foot and ankle are acceptable because non–weight-bearing radiographs are often misleading.[51–53] Furthermore, the standing position may help to standardize the radiograph technique, allowing more reliable comparison of interindividual and intraindividual radiographs. The ankle alignment should be analyzed and evaluated on all 3 levels: supramalleolar, intra-articular, and inframalleolar. The supramalleolar ankle alignment (**Fig. 3**) should be assessed in the coronal and sagittal planes by measurement of the medial distal tibial angle and anterior distal tibial angle (**Fig. 4**), respectively.[54,55] The anterior distal tibial angle has been measured as 83.0° ± 3.6° (range, 76°–97°).[55] The medial distal tibial angle has been measured as 92.4° ± 3.1° (range, 88°–100°) in a radiographic study[54] and 93.3° ± 3.2° (range, 88°–100°) in a cadaver

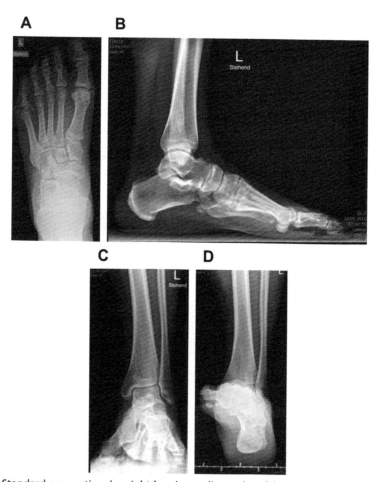

Fig. 2. Standard conventional weight-bearing radiographs of foot and ankle. (*A*) Anteroposterior and (*B*) lateral views of the foot, (*C*) mortise view of the ankle, and (*D*) Saltzman view of the hindfoot.

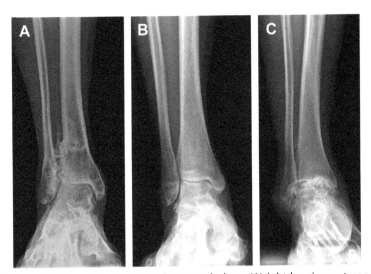

Fig. 3. Supramalleolar ankle alignment in coronal plane. Weight-bearing anteroposterior ankle radiographs showing (*A*) valgus alignment, (*B*) normal alignment, and (*C*) varus alignment in the coronal plane. (*From* Barg A, Knupp M, Henninger HB, et al. Total ankle replacement using HINTEGRA, an unconstrained, three-component system: surgical technique and pitfalls. Foot Ankle Clin 2012;17(4):610; with permission.)

study.[54,56] The measurement of the medial distal tibial angle depends on radiograph technique; it is not the same on whole-leg images and mortise views of the ankle.[57] In another radiographic study, a substantial disagreement in the medial distal angle, with differences up to 12°, was found between the mortise and Saltzman views.[58]

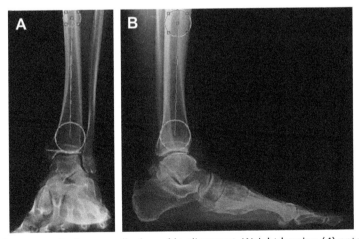

Fig. 4. Measurement of supramalleolar ankle alignment. Weight-bearing (*A*) anteroposterior and (*B*) lateral views of the ankle of a 51-year-old male patient showing the measurement of medial distal tibial angle[57] (in this case 87°) and the measurement of anterior distal tibial angle[55] (in this case 84°). (*From* Barg A, Knupp M, Henninger HB, et al. Total ankle replacement using HINTEGRA, an unconstrained, three-component system: surgical technique and pitfalls. Foot Ankle Clin 2012;17(4):611; with permission.)

Therefore, the authors generally recommend measurement of the medial distal tibial angle using only the mortise view. The Saltzman view[50] should be used to assess the inframalleolar alignment. Different measurement techniques can be applied to quantify the inframalleolar hindfoot alignment (**Fig. 5**).[59] First, the angle between the longitudinal axis of the tibia and the calcaneal axis can be measured as suggested by Cobey[60] and Reilingh and colleagues.[61] Another radiographic measurement addresses the angles between the longitudinal axis of the tibia and lines adapted to the medial and lateral osseous contour of the calcaneus, as described by Donovan and Rosenberg.[62] Finally, the apparent moment arm can be measured as the distance of the most distal point of the plantar calcaneal contour to the tibial shaft axis as originally described by Saltzman and el Khoury.[50] Buck and colleagues[59] addressed the rotational stability of the aforementioned measurement techniques using the Saltzman view, and demonstrated that the method described by Donovan and Rosenberg[62] has the highest reliability.

In most patients presenting with ankle OA, the authors perform single-photon emission computed tomography/computed tomography (SPECT-CT) to evaluate the extent of degenerative changes and their biological activities (**Fig. 6**). This radiographic modality may also help to assess the osteoarthritic changes in the neighboring joints of the hindfoot and midfoot, where the number and configuration of joints are very complex.[63] Pagenstert and colleagues[63] have demonstrated that SPECT-CT has significantly higher interobserver and intraobserver reliability than measurement using CT alone or CT and bone scanning together. Knupp and

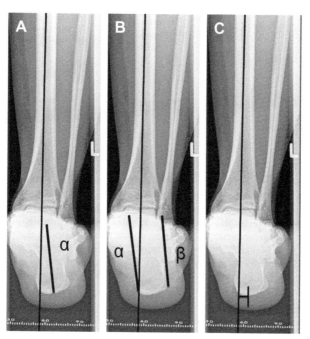

Fig. 5. Different measurement techniques of the inframalleolar hindfoot alignment. (*A*) Angle between the longitudinal axis of the tibia and the calcaneal axis. (*B*) Angles between the longitudinal axis of the tibia and lines adapted to the medial and lateral osseous contour of the calcaneus. (*C*) Distance of the most distal point of the plantar calcaneal contour to the tibial shaft axis.

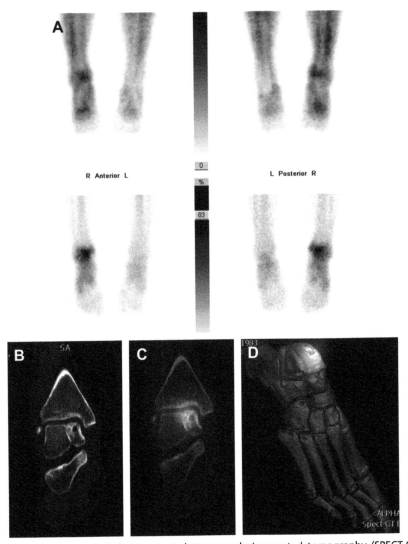

Fig. 6. Single-photon emission computed tomography/computed tomography (SPECT-CT). (*A*) Scintigraphy shows increased enhancement of technetium-99m dicarboxypropane-diphosphonic acid. However, the exact localization of lesion in the tibiotalar joint is not possible because of low resolution. (*B*) CT scan shows cystic lesion on the medial shoulder of the talus. (*C*) SPECT-CT combines information of both previously mentioned diagnostic modalities, showing biological activity of the cystic lesion. (*D*) Three-dimensional reconstruction may allow easier and better analysis and understanding of lesion localization.

colleagues[64] used weight-bearing radiographs, conventional CT, bone scintigraphy, and SPECT-CT in patients with valgus or varus ankle OA. On the SPECT-CT images the varus malaligned ankles showed significantly higher radioisotope uptake in the medial joint compartment than in the lateral one. By contrast, the valgus malaligned ankles showed significantly greater uptake in the lateral areas than in the medial regions. The results of this study showed that SPECT-CT is a unique radiographic tool, allowing the simultaneous analysis of the morphology and metabolism of

Table 3
Ankle osteoarthritis classification system (as suggested by Takakura and colleagues[19,69])

Stage	Radiographic Osteoarthritis Signs
Stage 1	No joint-space narrowing, but early sclerosis and osteophyte formation
Stage 2	Narrowing of the joint space medially
Stage 3	Obliteration of the joint space with subchondral bone contact medially
Stage 4	Obliteration of the whole joint space with complete bone contact

Adapted from Takakura Y, Tanaka Y, Kumai T, et al. Low tibial osteotomy for osteoarthritis of the ankle. Results of a new operation in 18 patients. J Bone Joint Surg Br 1995;77(1):50; and Takakura Y, Tanaka Y, Sugimoto K. The treatment for osteoarthritis of the ankle joint. Jpn J Rheum Joint Surg 1986;1986:348.

degenerative changes of the tibiotalar joint and hindfoot alignment.[64] Kretzschmar and colleagues[65] performed a prospective study to address the feasibility and to investigate the predictive value of SPECT-CT for image-guided diagnostic infiltration in 30 participants with chronic foot pain. In total, 27 of 30 patients reported a significant pain reduction of 50% or more, as measured using VAS, resulting in a very high response rate of 90%.[65]

Magnetic resonance imaging (MRI) has evolved to become a very helpful diagnostic tool, allowing evaluation of cartilage and periarticular soft tissues and tendons around the ankle joint.[66] Different anatomic variants should be considered at the evaluation of MRI.[67] The authors suggest performing high-quality 3-T MRI with 1-mm slices, as this method provides double the signal-to-noise ratio as 1.5-T MRI, thus shortening the imaging time and improving image quality.[68]

ANKLE OSTEOARTHRITIS CLASSIFICATION SYSTEM

Takakura and colleagues[19,69] used weight-bearing radiographs to classify ankle OA into 4 stages (**Table 3**). For clinical use the investigators simplified the classification, describing stage 1 as early, stages 2 and 3 as intermediate, and stage 4 as late.[19,69] Tanaka and colleagues[70] slightly modified the Takakura classification as follows. Stage 1: early sclerosis and formation of osteophytes without narrowing of the joint space; Stage 2: narrowing of the medial joint space; Stage 3A: obliteration of the medial joint space with subchondral bone contact limited to the medial malleolus; Stage 3B: subchondral bone contact extending to the roof of the dome of the talus; and Stage 4: obliteration of the entire joint space, resulting in bone contact throughout the ankle.

Table 4
Ankle osteoarthritis classification system (as suggested by Giannini and colleagues[71])

Stage	Radiographic Osteoarthritis Signs
Stage 0	Normal joint or subchondral sclerosis
Stage 1	Presence of osteophytes without joint-space narrowing
Stage 2	Joint-space narrowing with or without osteophytes
Stage 3	Subtotal or total disappearance or deformation of joint space

Adapted from Giannini S, Buda R, Faldini C, et al. The treatment of severe posttraumatic arthritis of the ankle joint. J Bone Joint Surg Am 2007;89 Suppl 3:15.

Table 5
Ankle osteoarthritis classification system based on weight-bearing radiographs (as suggested by Cheng and colleagues[13])

Stage	Radiographic Osteoarthritis Signs
Stage 0	No reduction of the joint space Normal alignment
Stage 1	Slight reduction of the joint space Slight formation of deposits at the joint margins Normal alignment
Stage 2	More pronounced change than mentioned above Subchondral osseous sclerotic configuration Mild malalignment
Stage 3	Joint space reduced to about half the height of the uninjured side Rather pronounced formation of deposits Obvious varus or valgus alignment
Stage 4	Joint space has completely or practically disappeared

Adapted from Cheng YM, Huang PJ, Hong SH, et al. Low tibial osteotomy for moderate ankle arthritis. Arch Orthop Trauma Surg 2001;121(6):355.

The ankle OA classification system as suggested by Giannini and colleagues[71] is similar that of Takakura and is based on radiographic evaluation of degenerative changes of the tibiotalar joint (eg, presence of osteophytes or narrowing of joint space) (**Table 4**).

A similar classification has been used by Cheng and colleagues,[13] which is a modified Cedell[72] classification (**Table 5**). These investigators classified degree 1 as mild OA, degrees 2 and 3 as moderate, and degree 4 as severe OA. Harstall and colleagues[15] used a simple classification of osteoarthritic changes in the ankle as suggested by van Dijk and colleagues[73]: Grade 0, normal joint or subchondral sclerosis; Grade I, osteophytes without joint-space narrowing; Grade II, joint-space narrowing with or without osteophytes; Grade III, (sub)total disappearance or deformation of the joint space.

Recently, Krause and colleagues[74] described a novel classification system, the Canadian Orthopedic Foot and Ankle Society (COFAS) classification (**Table 6**), and investigated its interobserver and intraobserver reliability.

Table 6
COFAS classification system for end-stage ankle osteoarthritis (as suggested by Krause and colleagues[74])

Type	Description
Type 1	Isolated ankle arthritis
Type 2	Ankle arthritis with intra-articular varus or valgus deformity or a tight heel cord, or both
Type 3	Ankle arthritis with hindfoot deformity, tibial malunion, midfoot abductus or adductus, supinated midfoot, plantarflexed first ray, etc
Type 4	Types 1–3 plus subtalar, calcaneocuboid, or talonavicular arthritis

Adapted from Krause FG, Di Silvestro M, Penner MJ, et al. The postoperative COFAS end-stage ankle arthritis classification system: interobserver and intraobserver reliability. Foot Ankle Spec 2012;5(1):32.

SUMMARY

Ankle OA is less common than OA of the other major joints of the lower extremity (knee or hip). However, the clinical importance of ankle OA should not be underestimated. Patients with ankle OA have a lower quality of life and substantial functional limitations.[4,32] Unlike the hip and knee joint, the ankle joint is often affected by posttraumatic OA.[5,6] The diagnosis of osteoarthritic ankle joint starts with clinical assessment, and includes assessment of alignment and stability and measurement of range of motion. Different radiographic modalities may help to recognize and analyze the underlying reasons for ankle OA. Only weight-bearing radiographs of the foot and ankle should be performed. Additional imaging modalities such as MRI and SPECT-CT may help to evaluate the extent of degenerative changes and their biological activities. The current ankle OA classification systems are based on radiographic evaluation of degenerative changes of the tibiotalar joint.

REFERENCES

1. Buckwalter JA, Martin JA. Osteoarthritis. Adv Drug Deliv Rev 2006;58(2):150–67.
2. Buckwalter JA, Saltzman C, Brown T. The impact of osteoarthritis: implications for research. Clin Orthop Relat Res 2004;(Suppl 427):S6–15.
3. Reginster JY. The prevalence and burden of arthritis. Rheumatology (Oxford) 2002;41(Supp 1):3–6.
4. Glazebrook M, Daniels T, Younger A, et al. Comparison of health-related quality of life between patients with end-stage ankle and hip arthrosis. J Bone Joint Surg Am 2008;90(3):499–505.
5. Valderrabano V, Horisberger M, Russell I, et al. Etiology of ankle osteoarthritis. Clin Orthop Relat Res 2009;467(7):1800–6.
6. Saltzman CL, Salamon ML, Blanchard GM, et al. Epidemiology of ankle arthritis: report of a consecutive series of 639 patients from a tertiary orthopaedic center. Iowa Orthop J 2005;25:44–6.
7. Thomas RH, Daniels TR. Ankle arthritis. J Bone Joint Surg Am 2003;85-A(5): 923–36.
8. Daniels T, Thomas R. Etiology and biomechanics of ankle arthritis. Foot Ankle Clin 2008;13(3):341–52.
9. Hintermann B. Characteristics of the diseased ankle. In: Hintermann B, editor. Total ankle arthroplasty: historical overview, current concepts and future perspectives. Wien (Austria), New York: Springer; 2005. p. 5–9.
10. Brown TD, Johnston RC, Saltzman CL, et al. Posttraumatic osteoarthritis: a first estimate of incidence, prevalence, and burden of disease. J Orthop Trauma 2006;20(10):739–44.
11. Valderrabano V, Hintermann B, Horisberger M, et al. Ligamentous posttraumatic ankle osteoarthritis. Am J Sports Med 2006;34(4):612–20.
12. Frey C, Zamora J. The effects of obesity on orthopaedic foot and ankle pathology. Foot Ankle Int 2007;28(9):996–9.
13. Cheng YM, Huang PJ, Hong SH, et al. Low tibial osteotomy for moderate ankle arthritis. Arch Orthop Trauma Surg 2001;121(6):355–8.
14. Lee WC, Moon JS, Lee K, et al. Indications for supramalleolar osteotomy in patients with ankle osteoarthritis and varus deformity. J Bone Joint Surg Am 2011;93(13):1243–8.
15. Harstall R, Lehmann O, Krause F, et al. Supramalleolar lateral closing wedge osteotomy for the treatment of varus ankle arthrosis. Foot Ankle Int 2007; 28(5):542–8.

16. Neumann HW, Lieske S, Schenk K. Supramalleolar, subtractive valgus osteotomy of the tibia in the management of ankle joint degeneration with varus deformity. Oper Orthop Traumatol 2007;19(5–6):511–26 [in German].

17. Pagenstert GI, Hintermann B, Barg A, et al. Realignment surgery as alternative treatment of varus and valgus ankle osteoarthritis. Clin Orthop Relat Res 2007; 462:156–68.

18. Pagenstert G, Knupp M, Valderrabano V, et al. Realignment surgery for valgus ankle osteoarthritis. Oper Orthop Traumatol 2009;21(1):77–87.

19. Takakura Y, Tanaka Y, Kumai T, et al. Low tibial osteotomy for osteoarthritis of the ankle. Results of a new operation in 18 patients. J Bone Joint Surg Br 1995; 77(1):50–4.

20. Takakura Y, Takaoka T, Tanaka Y, et al. Results of opening-wedge osteotomy for the treatment of a post-traumatic varus deformity of the ankle. J Bone Joint Surg Am 1998;80(2):213–8.

21. McKinley TO, Rudert MJ, Koos DC, et al. Incongruity versus instability in the etiology of posttraumatic arthritis. Clin Orthop Relat Res 2004;423:44–51.

22. McKinley TO, Rudert MJ, Koos DC, et al. Pathomechanic determinants of post-traumatic arthritis. Clin Orthop Relat Res 2004;(Suppl 427):S78–88.

23. Horisberger M, Valderrabano V, Hintermann B. Posttraumatic ankle osteoarthritis after ankle-related fractures. J Orthop Trauma 2009;23(1):60–7.

24. Lübbeke A, Salvo D, Stern R, et al. Risk factors for post-traumatic osteoarthritis of the ankle: an eighteen year follow-up study. Int Orthop 2012;36(7):1403–10.

25. Stufkens SA, Knupp M, Horisberger M, et al. Cartilage lesions and the development of osteoarthritis after internal fixation of ankle fractures: a prospective study. J Bone Joint Surg Am 2010;92(2):279–86.

26. McKinley TO, Tochigi Y, Rudert MJ, et al. The effect of incongruity and instability on contact stress directional gradients in human cadaveric ankles. Osteoarthritis Cartilage 2008;16(11):1363–9.

27. Tochigi Y, Rudert MJ, McKinley TO, et al. Correlation of dynamic cartilage contact stress aberrations with severity of instability in ankle incongruity. J Orthop Res 2008;26(9):1186–93.

28. Anderson DD, Van Hofwegen C, Marsh JL, et al. Is elevated contact stress predictive of post-traumatic osteoarthritis for imprecisely reduced tibial plafond fractures? J Orthop Res 2011;29(1):33–9.

29. Tochigi Y, Buckwalter JA, Martin JA, et al. Distribution and progression of chondrocyte damage in a whole-organ model of human ankle intra-articular fracture. J Bone Joint Surg Am 2011;93(6):533–9.

30. Marsh JL, Buckwalter J, Gelberman R, et al. Articular fractures: does an anatomic reduction really change the result? J Bone Joint Surg Am 2002; 84-A(7):1259–71.

31. Egloff C, Huegle T, Valderrabano V. Biomechanics and pathomechanisms of osteoarthritis. Swiss Med Wkly 2012;142:w13583.

32. Segal AD, Shofer J, Hahn ME, et al. Functional limitations associated with end-stage ankle arthritis. J Bone Joint Surg Am 2012;94(9):777–83.

33. Ingrosso S, Benedetti MG, Leardini A, et al. GAIT analysis in patients operated with a novel total ankle prosthesis. Gait Posture 2009;30(2):132–7.

34. Piriou P, Culpan P, Mullins M, et al. Ankle replacement versus arthrodesis: a comparative gait analysis study. Foot Ankle Int 2008;29(1):3–9.

35. Valderrabano V, Nigg BM, von TV, et al. Gait analysis in ankle osteoarthritis and total ankle replacement. Clin Biomech (Bristol, Avon) 2007;22(8):894–904.

36. Huskisson EC. Measurement of pain. Lancet 1974;2(7889):1127–31.

37. Barg A, Elsner A, Hefti D, et al. Haemophilic arthropathy of the ankle treated by total ankle replacement: a case series. Haemophilia 2010;16(4):647–55.
38. Barg A, Elsner A, Hefti D, et al. Total ankle arthroplasty in patients with hereditary hemochromatosis. Clin Orthop Relat Res 2010;469(5):1427–35.
39. Buck P, Morrey BF, Chao EY. The optimum position of arthrodesis of the ankle. A gait study of the knee and ankle. J Bone Joint Surg Am 1987;69(7):1052–62.
40. Saltzman CL, Nawoczenski DA, Talbot KD. Measurement of the medial longitudinal arch. Arch Phys Med Rehabil 1995;76(1):45–9.
41. Frigg A, Nigg B, Davis E, et al. Does alignment in the hindfoot radiograph influence dynamic foot-floor pressures in ankle and tibiotalocalcaneal fusion? Clin Orthop Relat Res 2010;468(12):3362–70.
42. Valderrabano V, Nigg BM, von TV, et al. J. Leonard Goldner Award 2006. Total ankle replacement in ankle osteoarthritis: an analysis of muscle rehabilitation. Foot Ankle Int 2007;28(2):281–91.
43. Valderrabano V, von TV, Nigg BM, et al. Lower leg muscle atrophy in ankle osteoarthritis. J Orthop Res 2006;24(12):2159–69.
44. Barg A, Elsner A, Anderson AE, et al. The effect of three-component total ankle replacement malalignment on clinical outcome: pain relief and functional outcome in 317 consecutive patients. J Bone Joint Surg Am 2011;93(21): 1969–78.
45. Hintermann B, Barg A, Knupp M, et al. Conversion of painful ankle arthrodesis to total ankle arthroplasty. J Bone Joint Surg Am 2009;91(4):850–8.
46. Lindsjö U, Danckwardt-Lilliestrom G, Sahlstedt B. Measurement of the motion range in the loaded ankle. Clin Orthop Relat Res 1985;199(199):68–71.
47. Coetzee JC, Castro MD. Accurate measurement of ankle range of motion after total ankle arthroplasty. Clin Orthop Relat Res 2004;424(424):27–31.
48. Hintermann B, Valderrabano V, Dereymaeker G, et al. The HINTEGRA ankle: rationale and short-term results of 122 consecutive ankles. Clin Orthop Relat Res 2004;424(424):57–68.
49. Pagenstert GI, Hintermann B, Knupp M. Operative management of chronic ankle instability: plantaris graft. Foot Ankle Clin 2006;11(3):567–83.
50. Saltzman CL, el Khoury GY. The hindfoot alignment view. Foot Ankle Int 1995; 16(9):572–6.
51. Min W, Sanders R. The use of the mortise view of the ankle to determine hindfoot alignment: technique tip. Foot Ankle Int 2010;31(9):823–7.
52. Hunt MA, Birmingham TB, Jenkyn TR, et al. Measures of frontal plane lower limb alignment obtained from static radiographs and dynamic gait analysis. Gait Posture 2008;27(4):635–40.
53. Ellis SJ, Deyer T, Williams BR, et al. Assessment of lateral hindfoot pain in acquired flatfoot deformity using weightbearing multiplanar imaging. Foot Ankle Int 2010;31(5):361–71.
54. Knupp M, Ledermann H, Magerkurth O, et al. The surgical tibiotalar angle: a radiologic study. Foot Ankle Int 2005;26(9):713–6.
55. Magerkurth O, Knupp M, Ledermann H, et al. Evaluation of hindfoot dimensions: a radiological study. Foot Ankle Int 2006;27(8):612–6.
56. Inman VT. The joints of the ankle. Baltimore (MD): Williams & Wilkins; 1976.
57. Stufkens SA, Barg A, Bolliger L, et al. Measurement of the medial distal tibial angle. Foot Ankle Int 2011;32:288–93.
58. Barg A, Harris MD, Henninger HB, et al. Medial distal tibial angle: comparison between weightbearing mortise view and hindfoot alignment view. Foot Ankle Int 2012;33(8):655–61.

59. Buck FM, Hoffmann A, Mamisch-Saupe N, et al. Hindfoot alignment measurements: rotation-stability of measurement techniques on hindfoot alignment view and long axial view radiographs. AJR Am J Roentgenol 2011;197(3): 578–82.

60. Cobey JC. Posterior roentgenogram of the foot. Clin Orthop Relat Res 1976;118: 202–7.

61. Reilingh ML, Beimers L, Tuijthof GJ, et al. Measuring hindfoot alignment radiographically: the long axial view is more reliable than the hindfoot alignment view. Skeletal Radiol 2010;39(11):1103–8.

62. Donovan A, Rosenberg ZS. Extraarticular lateral hindfoot impingement with posterior tibial tendon tear: MRI correlation. AJR Am J Roentgenol 2009; 193(3):672–8.

63. Pagenstert GI, Barg A, Leumann AG, et al. SPECT-CT imaging in degenerative joint disease of the foot and ankle. J Bone Joint Surg Br 2009;91(9):1191–6.

64. Knupp M, Pagenstert GI, Barg A, et al. SPECT-CT compared with conventional imaging modalities for the assessment of the varus and valgus malaligned hindfoot. J Orthop Res 2009;27(11):1461–6.

65. Kretzschmar M, Wiewiorski M, Rasch H, et al. ^{99m}Tc-DPD-SPECT/CT predicts the outcome of imaging-guided diagnostic anaesthetic injections: a prospective cohort study. Eur J Radiol 2011;80(3):e410–5.

66. Haygood TM. Magnetic resonance imaging of the musculoskeletal system: part 7. The ankle. Clin Orthop Relat Res 1997;336(336):318–36.

67. Gyftopoulos S, Bencardino JT. Normal variants and pitfalls in MR imaging of the ankle and foot. Magn Reson Imaging Clin N Am 2010;18(4):691–705.

68. Chhabra A, Soldatos T, Chalian M, et al. Current concepts review: 3T magnetic resonance imaging of the ankle and foot. Foot Ankle Int 2012;33(2):164–71.

69. Takakura Y, Aoki T, Sugimoto K, et al. The treatment for osteoarthritis of the ankle joint. Jpn J Joint Dis 1986;5:347–52.

70. Tanaka Y, Takakura Y, Hayashi K, et al. Low tibial osteotomy for varus-type osteoarthritis of the ankle. J Bone Joint Surg Br 2006;88(7):909–13.

71. Giannini S, Buda R, Faldini C, et al. The treatment of severe posttraumatic arthritis of the ankle joint. J Bone Joint Surg Am 2007;89(Suppl 3):15–28.

72. Cedell CA. Outward rotation-supination injuries of the ankle. Clin Orthop Relat Res 1965;42:97–100.

73. van Dijk CN, Verhagen RA, Tol JL. Arthroscopy for problems after ankle fracture. J Bone Joint Surg Br 1997;79(2):280–4.

74. Krause FG, Di Silvestro M, Penner MJ, et al. The postoperative COFAS end-stage ankle arthritis classification system: interobserver and intraobserver reliability. Foot Ankle Spec 2012;5(1):31–6.

Biomechanics of Asymmetric Ankle Osteoarthritis and Its Joint-Preserving Surgery

Corina Nüesch, PhD[a],*, Alexej Barg, MD[b], Geert I. Pagenstert, MD[b], Victor Valderrabano, MD, PhD[a,b],*

KEYWORDS

- Biomechanics • Electromyography • Gait analysis • Osteoarthritis
- Supramalleolar osteotomies

KEY POINTS

- The hindfoot alignment has no influence on walking speed and step length.
- Patients with asymmetric ankle osteoarthritis have a significantly lower hindfoot range of motion, ankle plantarflexion moment, and ankle joint power during walking than healthy subjects.
- The hindfoot alignment influences the timing and intensity of the activation of the lower leg muscles.
- After realignment surgery, the patients still have a lower hindfoot range of motion, ankle plantarflexion moment, and ankle joint power than the contralateral side and healthy subjects.
- The temporal muscle activation of the lower leg muscles shows no differences to healthy subjects in patients after realignment surgery.

INTRODUCTION

Osteoarthritis (OA) of the ankle joint predominantly develops after trauma.[1,2] More than half of the patients have a malalignment of the hindfoot; more than half of the patients have varus ankle OA and less than 10% have valgus ankle OA.[2] Patients with such asymmetric ankle OA and partially intact articular cartilage can benefit from joint-preserving realignment surgery.[3–6] The aim of these supramalleolar osteotomies is to realign the ankle and improve the joint congruency.

Gait analyses have frequently been used to quantify changes in the functional biomechanics of the lower extremity during walking in patients with ankle OA and after surgical treatment with ankle arthrodesis or total ankle replacement.[7–15] To measure

[a] Osteoarthritis Research Center, University Hospital of Basel, University of Basel, Spitalstrasse 21, Basel 4031, Switzerland; [b] Orthopaedic Department, University Hospital of Basel, Spitalstrasse 21, Basel 4031, Switzerland
* Corresponding authors.
E-mail addresses: corina.nueesch@usb.ch; victor.valderrabano@usb.ch

Foot Ankle Clin N Am 18 (2013) 427–436
http://dx.doi.org/10.1016/j.fcl.2013.06.002
1083-7515/13/$ – see front matter © 2013 Elsevier Inc. All rights reserved.

the joint kinematics (ie, joint angles), several markers are placed on the skin, which capture the motion of different body segments (**Fig. 1**). In many studies the foot is modeled as a single segment, although that the anatomy of the foot is more complex. In recent years, several foot models have been developed that allow measuring the foot kinematics in more detail.[16–18] These models have in common that they measure the 3-dimensional kinematics of the hindfoot, forefoot, and hallux segments. Another possible measurement method to capture more detailed ankle joint motion is by fluoroscopy.[19,20] The combination of marker-based gait analysis with force plates that measure the ground reaction forces enables the calculation of the joint kinetics (eg, joint moments and joint power) through inverse dynamics.[21] In the case of ankle OA, mainly the peak internal ankle plantarflexion moment and the absorbed and generated ankle joint power were studied.[7,12,15,22]

Another important aspect of the joint biomechanics that is often neglected in gait analysis studies on ankle OA is the role and adaptation of the lower leg muscles. For knee OA, it has already been proposed that weakness of the knee-stabilizing muscles plays an important role in the pathogenesis of OA.[23] Muscle weakness is also present in ankle OA.[24] Furthermore, it has been demonstrated that in healthy subjects the foot posture can influence the muscle activation.[25,26] This article therefore focuses not only on biomechanical adaptations (joint kinematics and joint kinetics) in patients with asymmetric ankle OA but also on neuromuscular adaptations.

BIOMECHANICS OF A HEALTHY ANKLE DURING WALKING

During walking, healthy subjects use a range of motion of the ankle joint complex of around 30° to 10° dorsiflexion and 20° plantarflexion.[27] At initial contact the heel is in a neutral or slightly plantarflexed position, which is followed by a first plantarflexion motion during the loading response. Then, from about 10% to 50% of the gait cycle the ankle gradually dorsiflexes. To push off from the ground, the foot is plantarflexed again. The maximum plantarflexion angle of about 20° is reached at the time of toe off. During the swing phase the foot is dorsiflexed to achieve enough foot clearance (**Fig. 2**A).[27] With more detailed foot models, such as the Oxford foot model,[16] a similar pattern of motion as for the ankle joint complex in the sagittal plane is seen for the hindfoot (see **Fig. 2**B). However, it is not only the hindfoot that contributes to the plantarflexion and dorsiflexion motion of the ankle joint complex during walking, but also the forefoot (see **Fig. 2**C). Studies with bone pins further showed that both midfoot

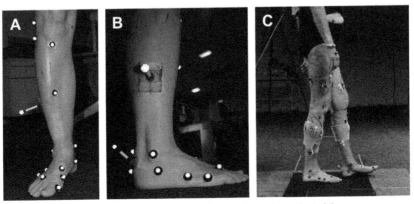

Fig. 1. Marker placement (*A, B*) and patient during the gait analysis (*C*).

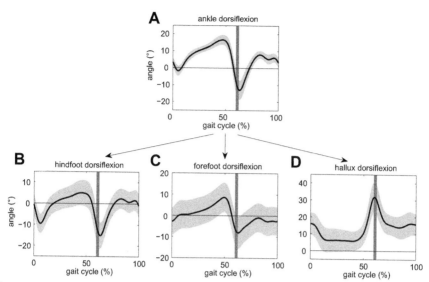

Fig. 2. Motion of the ankle joint complex (*A*), hindfoot (*B*), forefoot (*C*), and hallux (*D*) of healthy subjects in the sagittal plane during a gait cycle (starting and ending at heel strike). The light gray shaded area represents the mean ± SD. The dark gray vertical bars indicate the time of toe off. The hindfoot motion was measured with respect to the tibia, the forefoot motion with respect to the hindfoot, and the hallux motion with respect to the forefoot.

and forefoot add to the plantarflexion and dorsiflexion movement besides the main pronation and supination motion.[28,29] Additional measurements of the hallux motion showed that the main movement in the metatarsophalangeal-I joint occurs during toe off (see **Fig. 2**D).

BIOMECHANICAL ADAPTATIONS IN ASYMMETRIC ANKLE OA
Intra-articular Ankle Joint Biomechanics

The asymmetric alignment of the ankle joint leads to changes in the intra-articular pressure distribution and the contact area as demonstrated in studies with human lower leg cadavers. In the case of incongruent ankle joints (achieved by an additional osteotomy of the fibula), a varus alignment of the hindfoot leads a shift of the pressure in anteromedial direction and a reduction of the contact area. For a valgus alignment a pressure shift in posterolateral direction and a reduced contact area were observed.[30,31] However, in the specimens with an intact fibula and a congruent ankle joint, opposite changes were seen: 15° varus led to posterolateral pressure shifts and increased contact areas, while 15° valgus led to anteromedial pressure shifts and decreased contact areas.[30,31] These results indicate that in patients with asymmetric ankle OA a correction of the angle of the distal tibial joint surface alone might not be successful in re-establishing the physiologic load transfer in the ankle joint because the fibula, ligaments, and soft tissues might prevent the talus from following the correction of the tibia.[30–32]

Gait Biomechanics

Most gait analysis studies on patients with ankle OA did not report the alignment of the ankle joint in the frontal plane. One of the few results came from a large study that investigated the influence of the hindfoot alignment (varus, valgus, neutral) on the spatiotemporal gait parameters. There were no differences between the patient groups for the walking speed, step length, stride length, and stride width.[11] Similar results for the spatiotemporal gait parameters were also seen in another study with fewer patients (8 with varus and 4 with valgus ankle OA).[22] This study further investigated the force production and muscle activation of the patients with asymmetric ankle OA during walking. Compared with a group of healthy subjects, both patient groups had a lower peak ankle plantarflexion moment during push-off and generated less ankle power. However, it seemed that in the 4 patients with valgus ankle OA the peak ankle plantarflexion moment and ankle joint power were even lower than in the patients with varus ankle OA despite a comparable walking speed (**Fig. 3**).[22]

In general, gait analyses in patients with ankle OA revealed a lower walking speed, cadence, step length, and stride length than in healthy people of a similar age.[7,8] The patients also had reduced ranges of motion of the ankle joint complex,[7,12] as well as of the hindfoot, forefoot, and hallux segment[8,15] than either healthy subjects or the healthy contralateral limb. Although healthy persons had an ankle range of motion of about 30°, patients with ankle OA only had a range of motion of the ankle joint complex of about 20°.[7,12] Furthermore, the detailed foot kinematics during walking showed that the patients' hindfoot was excessively externally rotated throughout the gait cycle and that the varus motion of the forefoot during toe off was missing.[8] For the kinetics, lower peak ground reaction forces, peak ankle plantarflexion moment, and peak ankle joint power were measured on the osteoarthritic limb.[7,12,15] Compared with either the healthy contralateral side or the healthy subjects, the peak plantarflexion moment was reduced by about 15%, and the generated peak ankle joint power by between 25% and 50%.[7,12,15] In a fluoroscopy study, Kozanek and colleagues[19] showed that patients with ankle OA have a reduced motion of the tibiotalar joint during the first half of the stance phase and mainly of the subtalar joint during the second half of the stance phase. The motion of the subtalar joint was not only reduced compared with healthy control subjects but also pointed in the opposite direction. Although the subtalar joint of the healthy subjects had an internal rotation, plantarflexion, and inversion motion from mid-stance to toe off, this was changed in the ankle OA patients to external rotation, dorsiflexion, and eversion.[19] These results are in agreement with measurements from skin markers[8] and suggest that the normal motion coupling between the tibiotalar and subtalar joint did not exist in patients with ankle OA.[19]

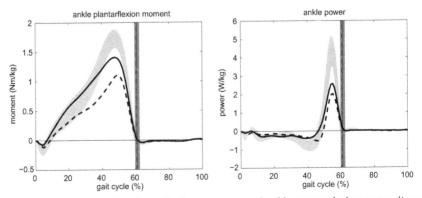

Fig. 3. Mean external ankle plantarflexion moment and ankle power during one gait cycle (start and end at heel strike) for patients with varus ankle OA (*solid line*) and with valgus ankle OA (*dashed line*). The vertical lines indicate the time of toe off. The gray shaded areas represent norm data (mean ± SD) from healthy controls for moment and power (*light gray area*) and time of toe off (*dark gray area*).

Neuromuscular Adaptations

Patients with ankle OA often experience muscle weakness and muscle atrophy, which also affects the joint biomechanics.[24,33] Muscle atrophy is associated with a lower calf circumference.[24] In patients with posttraumatic ankle OA, it was mainly the soleus muscle that had a reduced cross-sectional area in the magnetic resonance imaging.[33] These muscular adaptations not only cause muscle weakness but also alter the muscle activation patterns and intermuscular coordination of the lower leg muscles during isometric contractions and walking. It was seen that patients with end-stage ankle OA have a lower mean frequency of the electromyographic (EMG) signal during maximal isometric contractions for the tibialis anterior, gastrocnemius medialis, soleus, and peroneus longus muscle of the affected leg than both the contralateral leg and the healthy subjects.[24] For patients with early- to mid-stage asymmetric ankle OA, such spectral changes toward lower frequencies, were only found for the tibialis anterior muscle.[22] The meaning of these frequency shifts is still not entirely understood. In patients with OA, atrophy of fast-twitch type II muscle fibers is predominant.[34] Therefore, it was speculated that the higher amount of low-frequency content in the EMG signals is related to an atrophy of these type II fibers.[24,35]

During walking it was seen that the ankle OA patients have muscle activation patterns with broader activation regions for both legs compared with healthy controls. The differences in the activation patterns of the lower leg muscles in the affected leg were even distinct enough to allow a classification from those of the non-affected leg and healthy controls.[36] Furthermore, the EMG envelopes measured during walking had lower peaks for the patients than healthy controls (Nüesch C. unpublished data, 2013). In a small group of patients with early- to mid-stage varus and valgus ankle OA, the intermuscular coordination of the calf muscles was altered depending on the hindfoot alignment. Although in the healthy controls and the patients with varus ankle OA the gastrocnemius medialis muscle was maximally active before the gastrocnemius lateralis and soleus muscle, the opposite was the case for patients with valgus ankle OA.[22] Furthermore, the activation patterns of the peroneus longus muscle contained more low-frequency components in patients with valgus ankle OA than patients with varus ankle OA.[22] In healthy subjects with flat-arched feet the peroneus longus muscle was less active during push-off than in people with normal-arched feet.[25] Together with the lower muscle activation frequencies, this could indicate that the peroneus longus muscle was less active and produced less force in patients with a valgus hindfoot alignment than in patients with a varus hindfoot alignment.

BIOMECHANICS OF JOINT-PRESERVING SURGERIES
Gait Biomechanics

An important factor that influences the ankle joint biomechanics during walking is the ankle joint mobility. Although there is evidence that the passive plantar- and dorsiflexion range of motion increases after joint-preserving realignment surgery,[3,37,38] there are other studies that showed no change or even a slight decrease.[5,39] However, compared with healthy middle-aged people that have a passive ankle range of motion of about 70°,[40] the ankle range of motion of patients with ankle OA was reduced before and after surgery with values of around 35° to 50°.[3,5] Most studies used functional scores to assess the outcome of joint-preserving realignment surgeries. These scores often contain information about the ankle joint mobility or walking ability and showed an improvement after supramalleolar osteotomy.[3–6] Furthermore, patients had a higher sports and recreational activity level after surgery.[37]

First results on the gait biomechanics showed that patients followed a minimum of 3 years after surgery had a higher knee and hip flexion range of motion and tended to walk faster than patients with ankle OA.[41] However, the range of motion in hindfoot, forefoot, and hallux segments in plantar- and dorsiflexion was reduced compared with healthy subjects in both patients with ankle OA and patients following supramalleolar osteotomy (Nüesch C. unpublished data, 2013). Several years after surgery, patients had a higher hip flexion moment than patients with ankle OA, whereas the ankle plantarflexion moment did not change,[41] indicating that despite of the remaining limited ankle mobility, patients are able to walk faster after realignment surgery by increasing the motion of the hip and knee joint to facilitate the push-off from the floor and increase the step length. On the other hand, ranges of motion and peak joint moments increase with higher walking speeds.[42] The hip and knee range of motion and the peak hip flexion moment for the patients after realignment surgery were comparable to data from healthy subjects (Nüesch C. unpublished data, 2013). Hence, these changes could simply be effects of the higher walking speed and not indications of possible compensations and overload of other joints.

As **Fig. 4** shows, the joint angles between the different foot segments have similar shapes for all groups, healthy control subjects, affected leg, and nonaffected leg of the patients after surgery. The main difference was a reduced range of motion for the affected leg in the hindfoot dorsiflexion and hallux dorsiflexion angles. Such reduced ranges of motion of the ankle or hindfoot of the osteoarthritic limb were also seen after

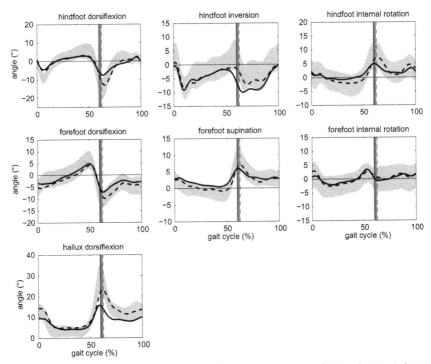

Fig. 4. Mean foot kinematics of 12 patients following a minimum of 1 year (range 1–9 years) after realignment surgery (*solid line*) in comparison to the nonaffected leg (*dashed line*) and healthy controls (*gray shaded area*: mean ± SD). The vertical lines indicate the time of toe off in the gait cycle for the affected leg (*solid*), nonaffected leg (*dashed*), and healthy controls (*dark gray area*).

ankle arthrodesis[13,43,44] or total ankle replacements.[7,13,45] Contrary to some results after ankle arthrodesis that showed an increased range of motion in the forefoot to compensate for the lack of motion in the hindfoot,[44] no such compensatory increase of forefoot or hallux motion was seen in these patients (see **Fig. 4**).

Neuromuscular Adaptations

To date there is still limited knowledge on the neuromuscular adaptations after surgical treatment of ankle OA. The ankle plantarflexion and dorsiflexion torques and thus the muscle strength increased after total ankle replacements but the spectral EMG changes (more low frequencies) remained.[46] For patients with valgus ankle OA changes in the timing of the peak calf muscle activation during walking were seen.[22] Preliminary data of 10 patients (5 patients with valgus ankle OA and 5 patients after realignment surgery for valgus ankle OA) showed improvements in the temporal activation of lower leg muscles.[47] In the patients with valgus ankle OA, the gastrocnemius medialis, soleus, and peroneus longus muscle were active during the whole stance phase, whereas these muscles were only active in the late stance phase for healthy control subjects and patients after realignment surgery. In addition, the patients with valgus ankle OA had a lower peak activation of the gastrocnemius medialis muscle and an earlier peak activation of the gastrocnemius lateralis muscle than the controls and postoperative patients.[47]

In a group of 7 asymmetric ankle OA patients that was measured around 8 years after realignment surgery (range 7–9 years) no significant differences for the temporal activation of the gastrocnemius medialis and lateralis, soleus, peroneus longus, and tibialis anterior muscle were found for the affected limb compared with healthy subjects (Nüesch C. unpublished data, 2013). **Fig. 5** shows that the peak activities of mainly the gastrocnemius lateralis and soleus muscle seemed to be lower for the affected limb compared with the contralateral healthy limb, but statistical analyses indicated no differences. However, generally the shape of the EMG envelopes of

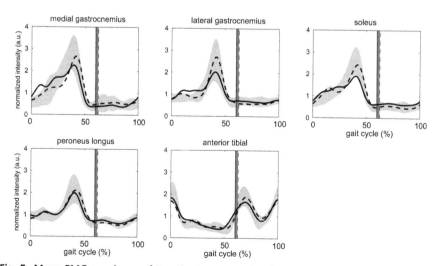

Fig. 5. Mean EMG envelopes of 7 patients measured at least 8 years after realignment surgery for the affected (*solid line*) and nonaffected leg (*dashed line*) compared to healthy controls (*gray shaded area*: mean ± SD). The vertical lines indicate the time of toe off in the gait cycle for the affected leg (*solid*), nonaffected leg (*dashed*), and healthy controls (*dark gray area*).

both legs of the postoperative patients corresponded well with the norm data for all 5 measured muscles.

SUMMARY

The results on the gait biomechanics in patients with asymmetric ankle OA showed that they have similar adaptations in their gait pattern as patients with end-stage ankle OA. The main observed changes in comparison with healthy subjects were as follows:

- A lower walking speed
- A lower ankle or hindfoot range of motion
- A lower peak ankle plantarflexion moment and lower peak ankle power
- A lower peak muscle activation of the calf muscles during walking

The treatment of asymmetric ankle OA by joint-preserving realignment surgery reduces the pain level and increases the patients' quality of life.[3–5] However, the gait patterns are highly influenced by the mobility of the ankle joint. Compared with healthy controls,[40] this ankle mobility remained often reduced after surgery, which explains the remaining reduction in the ranges of motion of the hindfoot. Despite the reduced hindfoot range of motion, the pattern of the hindfoot dorsiflexion angle during a gait cycle is comparable to the ones from healthy subjects (see **Fig. 4**). Generally one can therefore say that the gait patterns of patients after supramalleolar osteotomy were characterized by the following:

- A lower ankle or hindfoot range of motion than healthy subjects
- A lower peak ankle plantarflexion moment and lower peak ankle power than healthy subjects
- No differences in the temporal muscle activation compared with healthy subjects

There seem to be some improvements in the preferred walking speed after joint-preserving realignment surgery, but the biomechanical changes that were mainly related to the passive ankle range of motion remained. Nevertheless, the biomechanical and neuromuscular gait patterns of patients after supramalleolar osteotomies were comparable to those of patients with ankle OA and patients after total ankle replacement or ankle arthrodesis.

REFERENCES

1. Saltzman CL, Salamon ML, Blanchard GM, et al. Epidemiology of ankle arthritis: report of a consecutive series of 639 patients from a tertiary orthopaedic center. Iowa Orthop J 2005;25:44.
2. Valderrabano V, Horisberger M, Russell I, et al. Etiology of ankle osteoarthritis. Clin Orthop Relat Res 2009;467:1800.
3. Pagenstert GI, Hintermann B, Barg A, et al. Realignment surgery as alternative treatment of varus and valgus ankle osteoarthritis. Clin Orthop Relat Res 2007; 462:156.
4. Knupp M, Stufkens SA, Bolliger L, et al. Classification and treatment of supramalleolar deformities. Foot Ankle Int 2011;32:1023.
5. Tanaka Y, Takakura Y, Hayashi K, et al. Low tibial osteotomy for varus-type osteoarthritis of the ankle. J Bone Joint Surg Br 2006;88:909.
6. Lee WC, Moon JS, Lee K, et al. Indications for supramalleolar osteotomy in patients with ankle osteoarthritis and varus deformity. J Bone Joint Surg Am 2011; 93:1243.

7. Valderrabano V, Nigg BM, von Tscharner V, et al. Gait analysis in ankle osteoarthritis and total ankle replacement. Clin Biomech (Bristol, Avon) 2007;22:894.
8. Khazzam M, Long JT, Marks RM, et al. Preoperative gait characterization of patients with ankle arthrosis. Gait Posture 2006;24:85.
9. Barton T, Lintz F, Winson I. Biomechanical changes associated with the osteoarthritic, arthrodesed, and prosthetic ankle joint. Foot Ankle Surg 2011;17:52.
10. Brodsky JW, Polo FE, Coleman SC, et al. Changes in gait following the Scandinavian total ankle replacement. J Bone Joint Surg Am 2011;93:1890.
11. Queen RM, Carter JE, Adams SB, et al. Coronal plane ankle alignment, gait, and end-stage ankle osteoarthritis. Osteoarthritis Cartilage 2011;19:1338.
12. Segal AD, Shofer J, Hahn ME, et al. Functional limitations associated with end-stage ankle arthritis. J Bone Joint Surg Am 2012;94:777.
13. Piriou P, Culpan P, Mullins M, et al. Ankle replacement versus arthrodesis: a comparative gait analysis study. Foot Ankle Int 2008;29:3.
14. Hahn ME, Wright ES, Segal AD, et al. Comparative gait analysis of ankle arthrodesis and arthroplasty: initial findings of a prospective study. Foot Ankle Int 2012; 33:282.
15. Nüesch C, Valderrabano V, Huber C, et al. Gait patterns of asymmetric ankle osteoarthritis patients. Clin Biomech (Bristol, Avon) 2012;27:613.
16. Stebbins J, Harrington M, Thompson N, et al. Repeatability of a model for measuring multi-segment foot kinematics in children. Gait Posture 2006;23:401.
17. Kidder SM, Abuzzahab FS Jr, Harris GF, et al. A system for the analysis of foot and ankle kinematics during gait. IEEE Trans Rehabil Eng 1996;4:25.
18. Leardini A, Benedetti MG, Berti L, et al. Rear-foot, mid-foot and fore-foot motion during the stance phase of gait. Gait Posture 2007;25:453.
19. Kozanek M, Rubash HE, Li G, et al. Effect of post-traumatic tibiotalar osteoarthritis on kinematics of the ankle joint complex. Foot Ankle Int 2009;30:734.
20. de Asla RJ, Wan L, Rubash HE, et al. Six DOF in vivo kinematics of the ankle joint complex: application of a combined dual-orthogonal fluoroscopic and magnetic resonance imaging technique. J Orthop Res 2006;24:1019.
21. Whittle MW. Clinical gait analysis: a review. Hum Mov Sci 1996;15:369.
22. Nüesch C, Huber C, Pagenstert G, et al. Muscle activation of patients suffering from asymmetric ankle osteoarthritis during isometric contractions and level walking—a time-frequency analysis. J Electromyogr Kinesiol 2012;22:939.
23. Hurley MV. The role of muscle weakness in the pathogenesis of osteoarthritis. Rheum Dis Clin North Am 1999;25:283.
24. Valderrabano V, von Tscharner V, Nigg BM, et al. Lower leg muscle atrophy in ankle osteoarthritis. J Orthop Res 2006;24:2159.
25. Murley G, Menz H, Landorf K. Foot posture influences the electromyographic activity of selected lower limb muscles during gait. J Foot Ankle Res 2009;2:1.
26. Murley GS, Landorf KB, Menz HB, et al. Effect of foot posture, foot orthoses and footwear on lower limb muscle activity during walking and running: a systematic review. Gait Posture 2009;29:172.
27. Perry J. Gait analysis: normal and pathological function. Thorofare (NJ): Slack Inc; 1992.
28. Lundgren P, Nester C, Liu A, et al. Invasive in vivo measurement of rear-, mid-and forefoot motion during walking. Gait Posture 2008;28:93.
29. Nester CJ. Lessons from dynamic cadaver and invasive bone pin studies: do we know how the foot really moves during gait. J Foot Ankle Res 2009;2:18.
30. Stufkens SA, van Bergen CJ, Blankevoort L, et al. The role of the fibula in varus and valgus deformity of the tibia. J Bone Joint Surg Br 2011;93:1232.

31. Knupp M, Stufkens SA, van Bergen CJ, et al. Effect of supramalleolar varus and valgus deformities on the tibiotalar joint: a cadaveric study. Foot Ankle Int 2011; 32:609.

32. Knupp M, Hintermann B. Treatment of asymmetric arthritis of the ankle joint with supramalleolar osteotomies. Foot Ankle Int 2012;33:250.

33. Wiewiorski M, Dopke K, Steiger C, et al. Muscular atrophy of the lower leg in unilateral post traumatic osteoarthritis of the ankle joint. Int Orthop 2012;36:2079.

34. Fink B, Egl M, Singer J, et al. Morphologic changes in the vastus medialis muscle in patients with osteoarthritis of the knee. Arthritis Rheum 2007;56:3626.

35. Lyytinen T, Liikavainio T, Bragge T, et al. Postural control and thigh muscle activity in men with knee osteoarthritis. J Electromyogr Kinesiol 2010;20:1066.

36. von Tscharner V, Valderrabano V. Classification of multi muscle activation patterns of osteoarthritis patients during level walking. J Electromyogr Kinesiol 2010;20:676.

37. Pagenstert G, Leumann A, Hintermann B, et al. Sports and recreation activity of varus and valgus ankle osteoarthritis before and after realignment surgery. Foot Ankle Int 2008;29:985.

38. Cheng YM, Huang PJ, Hong SH, et al. Low tibial osteotomy for moderate ankle arthritis. Arch Orthop Trauma Surg 2001;121:355.

39. Takakura Y, Takaoka T, Tanaka Y, et al. Results of opening-wedge osteotomy for the treatment of a post-traumatic varus deformity of the ankle. J Bone Joint Surg Am 1998;80:213.

40. Soucie JM, Wang C, Forsyth A, et al. Range of motion measurements: reference values and a database for comparison studies. Haemophilia 2011;17:500.

41. Nüesch C, Huber C, Pagenstert G, et al. Asymmetric ankle osteoarthritis–long-term effects of realignment surgery on walking. In: Proceedings of the 20th Annual Meeting of the European Orthopaedics Research Society. Amsterdam (The Netherlands). Available at: http://www.eors2012.org/site/wp-content/uploads/2012/04/EORS20121.pdf. Accessed October 1, 2012.

42. Schwartz MH, Rozumalski A, Trost JP. The effect of walking speed on the gait of typically developing children. J Biomech 2008;41:1639.

43. Thomas R, Daniels TR, Parker K. Gait analysis and functional outcomes following ankle arthrodesis for isolated ankle arthritis. J Bone Joint Surg Am 2006;88:526.

44. Wu WL, Su FC, Cheng YM, et al. Gait analysis after ankle arthrodesis. Gait Posture 2000;11:54.

45. Ingrosso S, Benedetti MG, Leardini A, et al. GAIT analysis in patients operated with a novel total ankle prosthesis. Gait Posture 2009;30:132.

46. Valderrabano V, Nigg BM, von Tscharner V, et al. J. Leonard Goldner Award 2006. Total ankle replacement in ankle osteoarthritis: an analysis of muscle rehabilitation. Foot Ankle Int 2007;28:281.

47. Nüesch C, Pagenstert G, Huber C, et al. Muscle activation in valgus ankle osteoarthritis patients during walking—the effect of realignment surgery. In: Proceedings of the XIXth Congress of the International Society of Electrophysiology & Kinesiology. Brisbane (Australia): 2012.

Conservative Treatment of Asymmetric Ankle Osteoarthritis

Timo Schmid, MD, Fabian G. Krause, MD*

KEYWORDS

- Ankle • Arthritis • Nonoperative • Conservative • Treatment

KEY POINTS

- The evidence of conservative treatment of asymmetric ankle osteoarthritis in the literature is poor.
- Some data of conservative treatment measures including dietary supplementation, visco-supplementation, platelet-rich plasma, nonsteroidal anti-inflammatory drugs, corticosteroid injections, physical therapy, shoe modifications and orthoses, and patient's education in asymmetric ankle osteoarthritis is available.
- Reasonable success can be expected when conservative treatment is applied for asymmetric ankle osteoarthritis.
- Conservative treatment for at least 6 months is recommended for patients whose ankles do not qualify anymore for joint-preserving surgery and permanently for patients with medical or orthopedic contraindications for realignment surgery, total ankle replacement, and ankle arthrodesis.

INTRODUCTION

In the literature, there is a substantial lack of scientific reports and comparative studies on various conservative treatment options for asymmetric and global ankle osteoarthritis (OA). Because the evidence is poor, conservative treatment is frequently based on experience and patient preferences. Most therapies start with a combination of medications, orthoses, and shoe modifications.

Conservative treatment of asymmetric ankle OA is predominantly symptomatic and rarely causal. It is attempted generally as the initial treatment of ankle OA before any surgery for at least 6 months, to buy time in younger patients whose ankles do not anymore qualify for joint-preserving surgery and in patients with contraindications for joint-preserving surgery of the ankle, total ankle replacement (TAR), or ankle arthrodesis (AA). However, young and active patients with mild, moderate, and occasionally even advanced asymmetric ankle OA should be counseled that the

The authors have nothing to disclose.
Department of Orthopaedic Surgery, Inselspital, University of Berne, Freiburgstrasse, Berne 3010, Switzerland
* Corresponding author.
E-mail address: fabian.krause@insel.ch

postoperative outcome after joint-preserving realignment surgery (eg, supramalleolar osteotomy) might worsen over time when surgery is delayed (**Fig. 1**).

Successful conservative care is very dependent on the stage of the ankle OA and the patients' age and motivation. When choosing between conservative versus surgical treatment, the extent of subchondral bone exposed and the time over which the OA has advanced are factors that should be considered. Patients with only little exposition of subchondral bone and slow OA progression will likely respond better to conservative treatment.

This article summarizes the currently available (poor) evidence of conservative treatment of asymmetric ankle OA in the literature and adds the authors' experience with the particular technique.

Indications for conservative treatment of asymmetric ankle osteoarthritis as listed as follows:

- Initial treatment in the older patient for at least 6 months, before any surgery
- End-stage OA to buy time in the young and active patient
- Severe hindfoot instability that cannot be surgically stabilized
- Severe vascular or neurologic deficiency
- Neuropathic disorders (eg, Charcot foot)
- Unstable ankle and hindfoot soft tissues
- Ongoing infection of soft tissue, bone, or joint

Relative contraindication for conservative treatment of asymmetric ankle arthritis is as follows:

- Young and active patient with mild to moderate asymmetric ankle OA

DIETARY SUPPLEMENTATION

Glucosamine and chondroitin are the 2 supplementations that claim to have an affect on OA. Glucosamine is believed to restore and repair the extracellular matrix by acting

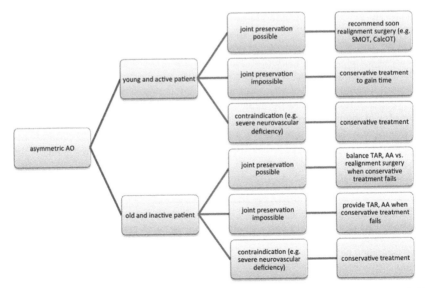

Fig. 1. Treatment algorithm for asymmetric ankle osteoarthritis. AO, ankle osteoarthritis; CalcOT, calcaneal osteotomyl; SMOT, supramalleolar osteotomy.

as a substrate for the formation of chondroitin sulfate and to stimulate the synovial production of hyaluronic acid.[1] Chondroitin sulfate seems to also initiate synovial fabrication of hyaluronic acid.[2]

Clinically a benefit of chondroitin or glucosamine for ankle OA is not yet proven. In knee OA a double-blind, placebo-controlled study showed a superiority of glucosamine over placebo,[3] whereas a *Cochrane Review*, which included 20 studies and 2570 patients, could not substantiate this superiority.[4] Although the authors do not discourage the use of these supplements, it is not a part of the authors' routine treatment program.

VISCOSUPPLEMENTATION

Hyaluronic acid injections are thought to help by its physical properties and by its anti-inflammatory, anabolic, and analgesic effects.[5] Similarly to the dietary supplementation, most literature about the effect of hyaluronic acid is published for knee OA. A new meta-analysis including 89 trials and 12,667 patients concluded that viscosupplementation in knee OA is associated with a small and clinically irrelevant benefit but increased risk for serious adverse events.[6]

In ankle OA viscosupplementation demonstrated evidence for significant improvement after 1 and 6 months of 5 weekly injections in a prospective randomized double-blind trial.[7] Similarly 3 weekly injections showed improvements in the Ankle Osteoarthritis Scale and American Orthopedic Foot and Ankle Society Hindfoot Score.[8] In contrast, a single injection of hyaluronic acid showed no difference to a saline solution.[9] A recent prospective clinical trial compared 3 weekly hyaluronic-acid injections to 6 weeks of exercise therapy. At 12-month follow-up, both groups showed significant pain relief and functional improvement, with no difference evident between groups.[10]

The role of viscosupplementation injections in the ankle joint remains controversial, with limited evidence to support their use. The effect of hyaluronic acid injections seems to be dose dependent and the ideal regimen of administration is not yet defined. The best patient for viscosupplementation should be younger than 65 years old and with mild ankle OA. The authors do not have experience in viscosupplementation.

PLATELET-RICH PLASMA

In the last decade, the application of platelet-rich plasma (PRP) has become increasingly popular in orthopedic surgery.[11] PRP is used for acceleration of bone healing, prevention, and treatment of soft-tissue and osseous infection, treatment of acute and chronic tendon or ligament injuries, and pain alleviation of osteoarthritic joints.[12–15]

As opposed to hyaluronic acid, PRP intra-articular injections seem to be more effective at relieving pain and improving motion in mild to moderate knee OA.[16] However, there is no evidence of the efficacy of PRP for ankle OA in the literature.

CORTICOSTEROID INJECTIONS

Intra-articular injections of corticosteroids are often used to decrease inflammation and pain.[17] Corticosteroids may have a role in the treatment of arthritic symptoms, but are not without risk. Due to their catabolic nature, routine injection can cause damage to the soft tissue envelope around the ankle joint and often success and effect duration decreases after several injections.

The efficacy of intra-articular corticosteroid injections in the osteoarthritic ankle has not been studied; most clinical studies have involved knee OA. The beneficial effects are often limited to a period of 8 weeks, with no difference between the effects of steroids and placebos over a longer time period.[18]

In a meta-analysis steroid injections resulted in a slightly longer and superior effect than systemic nonsteroid anti-inflammatory drugs (NSAIDs) in patients with knee OA, whereas no long-term effect was recorded.[19] In contrast another meta-analysis showed a benefit up to 16 to 24 weeks after injection of a dose equivalent to 50 mg prednisone.[20]

In the authors' experience the effect of corticosteroid injections into the ankle lasts for 4 to 8 weeks dependent on the extent of OA. An injection may not only be helpful for treatment to reduce inflammation but also provide useful information in the diagnostic process.[18] If the injection substantially reduces the individual's pain complaints, the authors are confident that the ankle is the primary source of pain. The authors do not like to give repeated injections of steroids because of the infection risk and catabolic risks to soft tissues (eg, local skin reactions such as depigmentation at the injection). To date, repeated corticosteroid injections seem to have no serious deleterious effect on articular cartilage.[21,22]

NONSTEROID ANTI-INFLAMMATORY DRUGS

Oral nonsteroidal anti-inflammatory medication should be temporarily incorporated into the initial phase of conservative treatment of ankle OA. NSAIDs reliably help to relieve the acute pain associated with OA and inflammation to some extent. Care must be exercised when prescribing these medications because of their known and sometimes substantial side effects and, if their long-term use is inevitably, patients should be carefully monitored.

There is no specific evidence about efficacy of NSAIDs in ankle OA in the literature but their value (and adverse side effects) has been proven in several level I arthritis studies. In the authors' experience, the efficacy of NSAIDs varies individually and diminishes over time.

PHYSICAL THERAPY

The implementation of exercises and physical activities can be a beneficial adjunct to patients' current pharmaceutical treatments and can help to increase muscle strength, motion, and endurance. Supervised physical therapy programs should focus on local anti-inflammatory measures, muscle strengthening, ankle and hindfoot joint mobilization to prevent joint stiffness, and gait education. Mobilization and strengthening exercises may decrease joint stress because dorsiflexion and plantarflexion muscle strength in individuals with ankle arthritis has been found to be decreased.[23]

Improvement of knee-cartilage glycosaminoglycan content, pain, and function in patients at risk of OA has been demonstrated in a prospective randomized Delayed Gadolinium Enhanced Magnetic Resonance Imaging of Cartilage magnetic resonance imaging study after moderate, supervised physical exercises.[24] Exercises may therefore also have important implications for disease prevention in patients at risk of developing ankle OA.

Occupational therapists may improve self-management strategies in patients with OA who experience difficulties at work.[25] To keep the patient independent during ambulation, it is important to prescribe gait training. As a result of the progressive nature of the OA, patients' activities of daily living are early impaired and they are oftentimes unable to hold their job. Occupational therapists can teach pacing (energy conservation), posture, and training of motor function and be helpful in choosing joint-protective orthoses.

Modalities such as electrical stimulation can be used for symptom management. The value of modalities in the long-term reduction of symptoms associated with post-traumatic ankle arthritis has not been well determined.

Thermotherapy includes a cold or hot source or a contrast bath with cold and hot water submersions. Local application of a cold (ice packs, ice chips, ice massage) or a hot (superficial heat, eg, hot packs, paraffin baths, and infrared, and deep heat, eg, electromagnetic waves and ultrasound) source can be used to provide short-term pain relief and to decrease joint stiffness.[25,26]

Therapeutic ultrasound carries high-frequency mechanical vibrations either in a continuous mode to alleviate pain by its thermal effects or by pulsed sequence to reduce inflammation. The heating effects of continuous ultrasound can also decrease muscle spasms and stimulate blood flow to help oppose inflammatory toxins.

To control pain and to increase muscle strength and function *electrotherapy* is applied for OA. In transcutaneous electrical nerve stimulation (TENS), electrical current is transmitted through electrodes to a specific muscle of interest to stimulate motor units.[25] TENS either transmits an electric current of high frequency with a low intensity for immediate pain relief or uses high-frequency burst impulses at a low intensity to relieve pain by stimulating pain-carrying fibers.[27]

Low-level laser therapy is another modality to treat pain and to improve function in patients with arthritis. The laser emits a single wavelength of pure light, which causes a photochemical reaction within the cell.[25]

There is no evidence of the efficacy of thermotherapy, therapeutic ultrasound, or TENS for ankle arthritis in the literature. However, the efficacy of these physical measures was substantially studied for rheumatoid patients and may also be applied to ankle arthritis originating from causes other than rheumatoid. Several reviews show that thermotherapy is more effective as an adjunct therapy than it is alone, whereas the effect of thermotherapy in isolation was rated unclear.[28–30] Randomized controlled trials (RCTs) showed low-quality evidence that ultrasound significantly decreases painful joints and increases function in rheumatoid patients and that the effects on pain outcomes applying TENS were conflicting.[28,31] For laser therapy 3 RCTs revealed significant improvements in pain and 2 RCTs found moderate evidence of increased ROM and flexibility.[32]

ORTHOSES AND SHOE MODIFICATION

Orthoses and shoe modifications can provide effective pain alleviation, provide improvement of life quality, and postpone TAR or AA in patients affected by advanced ankle arthritis with or without deformity.[33]

Because custom-made orthoses are expensive, off-the-shelf orthoses may be tried first to ascertain whether the patient will benefit from custom orthoses. Patients with rigid hindfoot deformities (eg, cavovarus feet) tolerate hard orthoses poorly. Commercially available inserts can be modified with cutouts, metatarsal pads, or foam rubber support according to the individual requirements. If the modified insert alleviates the discomfort substantially, a custom-made tridensity or semirigid orthosis is prescribed using the modified insert as a template.[34] A practical aspect of orthoses is the patient's compliance with the orthosis. Bulkiness, discomfort, and accessibility with shoe gear are factors that can contribute to patient apprehension.[33]

Because shoe wear modifications and bracing may not be cosmetically appealing and can restrict participation in activity, young individuals with posttraumatic ankle

OA are likely to be resistant to accept long-term shoe modifications and/or bracing as a treatment option.

As opposed to global ankle OA, asymmetric ankle OA allows unloading of the osteoarthritic side of the joint by shifting the load axis to the unaffected side with medial and lateral wedges or with realignment surgery (eg, lateralizing calcaneal osteotomy). Dependent on the arthritis stage, conservative treatment of ankle OA with orthoses and shoe modifications follows 2 biomechanical principles: (1) unloading of the osteoarthritic side of the ankle in the mild, moderate, and occasionally advanced stages with maintenance of ankle motion and (2) limitation and control of ankle motion and hindfoot stability in the advanced and end stages of OA.

If realignment surgery is not an option (see **Fig. 1**, algorithm), *shoe modifications* mainly include shock absorption and cushioning of the heel, application of a rocker bottom sole, and particularly in asymmetric ankle OA, medial and lateral wedges fixed inside or outside the shoe (**Fig. 2**). To prevent valgus decompensation of the hindfoot and midfoot or hindfoot varus instability with recurrent sprains, wedges incorporated in the insert or at the sole should not exceed 10 mm. Similarly to intra-articular blocks, the effect of these wedges also gives the patient and the surgeon an idea whether the patient will improve with realignment surgery by unloading the arthritic part of the joint.

The *rocker bottom sole* with a *cushioned heel* in a low shoe reduces impact at heel strike, transferring some sagittal plane motion from the ankle joint to the bottom of the shoe. Less rigid orthoses allow motion in the ankle and are indicated for mild to moderate ankle OA. Because older patients may be disturbed by gait instability, the rocker sole should be enough wide. Prefabricated low shoes and trainers are available (**Fig. 3**), but quality shoes can also be equipped subsequently with a rocker sole and heel cushion.

Even minimal motion within the advanced osteoarthritic ankle joint can elicit pain and limit weight-bearing and ambulation. The goal of more rigid or inflexible orthoses is therefore to control and limit ankle motion in the sagittal plane and to maintain the joint in plantigrade or neutral position. When considering bracing, there are many options, ranging from off-the-shelf lace-up-type athletic ankle braces to a custom-molded articulated (**Fig. 4**) or nonarticulated (**Fig. 5**) *ankle foot orthoses* (AFO) *high-top boots* with prefabricated lateral stabilization (**Fig. 6**), which are used to limit ankle motion.[35,36] Lace-up braces are easy to fit inside a shoe or a boot and offer stabilization comparable to plastic upright braces.[34] An Arizona brace (lace-up leather brace) provides superior ankle support while still fitting in many types of shoes, although the shoe needs to be bigger to accommodate the brace.

Direct comparisons of orthoses' designs in clinical trials are lacking but biomechanical studies have assessed the effect of designs on ankle and hindfoot motion.[37] A

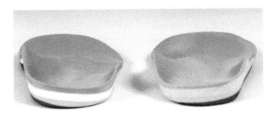

Fig. 2. Example of a medial heel wedge (*left*) and lateral heel wedge (*right*) of 5 mm incorporated in a right shoe insert. (*Courtesy of* Ortho-Team, Bern, Switzerland.)

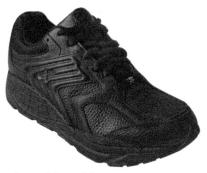

Fig. 3. Example of a low shoe with prefabricated rocker bottom sole and heel cushion. (*Courtesy of* Xelero AG, Zofingen, Switzerland; and Ortho-Team, Bern, Switzerland.)

rocker sole and solid-ankle cushion-heel were found to decrease ankle motion and aid in the transition from heel strike to push-off during level walking.[38] Three brace designs (custom-molded AFO, rigid hindfoot orthoses, and articulated hindfoot orthoses) were assessed for their efficacy to control and limit forefoot and hindfoot motion during walking in patients with ankle OA. The rigid hindfoot orthoses provided selective restriction of ankle–hindfoot motion while allowing sufficient forefoot motion compared with the custom-molded AFOs. The articulated hindfoot orthoses were ineffective in restricting hindfoot motion.[35] Custom foot orthoses and custom shoe gear led to a significant decrease in pain, increase in step length and stride length, and reduction in energy expenditure after 3 months of study.[39]

For mild to moderate asymmetric ankle OA, usually off-the-shelf or custom-made wedged inserts are started and a lace-up brace is added if symptoms are not adequately controlled and hindfoot instability is an issue. In the advanced arthritis cases, the use of a high-top boot with lateral stabilization (see **Fig. 6**) along with a rocker sole, heel cushion, and wedges (see **Fig. 2**) has worked the best.

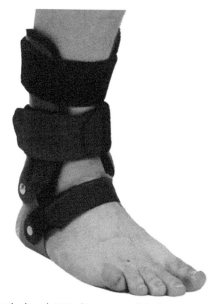

Fig. 4. Example of an articulated AFO. (*Courtesy of* Ortho-Team, Bern, Switzerland.)

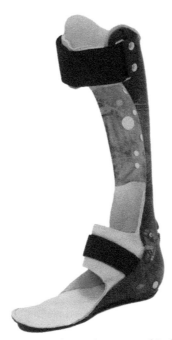

Fig. 5. Example of a high nonarticulated AFO. (*Courtesy of* Ortho-Team, Bern, Switzerland.)

PATIENT EDUCATION

Obesity consistently emerges as a potentially modifiable risk factor for the onset and progression of musculoskeletal disease. Obese patients should be counseled about the importance of losing weight. Weight loss decreases the reactive forces within the osteoarthritic joint and the risk of work-restricting musculoskeletal pain.[40] Moreover, it improves the effectiveness of both conservative and surgical options. Given the multifactorial nature of musculoskeletal disorders, it is likely that obesity may act as a permissive factor in ankle OA by interacting and potentiating the effects of

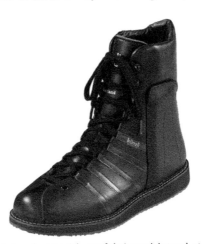

Fig. 6. Example of a high-top boot with prefabricated lateral stabilization. (*Courtesy of* Künzli-Swiss Shoe AG, Windisch, Switzerland; and Ortho-Team, Bern, Switzerland.)

other risk factors (eg, hindfoot malalignment).[41] However there is little scientific evidence directly linking musculoskeletal injury to altered biomechanics in the obese.

Although weight loss has been shown to potentially reduce pain[42] and improves the quality and quantity of cartilage in knee OA,[43] no such evidence exists for ankle OA. Nevertheless, patients with body mass index greater 25 have a 1.5 times higher risk for the diagnosis of foot and ankle OA.[44]

Activity modification and *avoidance of high-impact activities* must be discussed with the patients, while continuation and start of low-impact sports (eg, cycling and swimming) should be encouraged. Daily activities that are known to put high strain on the ankle (eg, climbing stairs) may need to be avoided. The use of a cane for ambulation offloads 25% of the body weight. Changing to a more sedentary job may make symptoms more manageable.[18]

DISCUSSION

The primary goal of conservative treatment of asymmetric ankle OA is pain alleviation. In the earlier OA stages this is succeeded biomechanically by unloading of the osteoarthritic side of the joint, whereas maintenance of ankle motion is desired or even improved with physiotherapy and exercises. In contrast, even little ankle motion can elicit pain in the advanced and end-stages of OA and is therefore limited and controlled by braces and boots. However, in cases of severe ankle and hindfoot instability (eg, due to neuropathic muscular imbalance), conservative treatment of asymmetric ankle OA also requires braces and high-top boots to stabilize the hindfoot but restricting ankle motion at the same time, even when the extent of OA is mild.

The evidence of conservative treatment in the management of individuals with asymmetric ankle OA is poorly defined. Some of the compiled literature had weak evidence because of limitations within its study. This indicates that further research is required to provide definitive conclusions on the use of the above-mentioned conservative treatments for asymmetric ankle OA. Other studies, whose conclusions can at least partially be adopted for ankle OA, had sufficient evidence to provide information to best treat patients with rheumatoid and knee arthritis, such as pharmacologic systemic and intra-articular therapy and custom-made foot orthoses, braces, and shoe modifications.

The authors' paradigm to direct the management from conservative to surgical intervention considers predominantly the patient's age, possible surgical preservation of the ankle joint, and medical or orthopedic contraindication for realignment surgery, TAR, and AA. Also the extent of exposed articular bone and the length of time over which the OA has developed need to be reflected. Individuals with large areas of exposed articular bone have poorer outcomes with conservative treatment than individuals with mild arthritic changes. Patients with an acute trauma and rapid onset of ankle OA seem to have poorer outcomes than those with chronic symptoms that occurred over several years.

A combination of different conservative methods seems to work better than any in isolation. At the authors' institution, the combination of NSAIDs, ankle support (eg, Künzli boot) with shoe inserts and modifications (eg, rocker bottom on the outside and heel wedges incorporated in the insert), and occasionally a corticosteroid injection are the measures that are currently used for conservative treatment of asymmetric ankle OA with reasonable success.

SUMMARY

The role and effectiveness for conservative treatment, such as medication, patient education, shoe modification, bracing, stretching, mobilization, strengthening, and symptom management, need to be further determined. There definitively is a place for conservative treatment with reasonable success in patients whose ankles do not qualify anymore for joint-preserving surgery and in patients with medical or orthopedic contraindications for realignment surgery, TAR, and AA.

REFERENCES

1. McCarty MF. Enhanced synovial production of hyaluronic acid may explain rapid clinical response to high-dose glucosamine in osteoarthritis. Med Hypotheses 1998;50:507–10.
2. Kato Y, Mukudai Y, Okimura A, et al. Effects of hyaluronic acid on the release of cartilage matrix proteoglycan and fibronectin from the cell matrix layer of chondrocyte cultures: interactions between hyaluronic acid and chondroitin sulfate glycosaminoglycan. J Rheumatol Suppl 1995;43:158–9.
3. Herrero-Beaumont G, Ivorra JA, Del Carmen Trabado M, et al. Glucosamine sulfate in the treatment of knee osteoarthritis symptoms: a randomized, double-blind, placebo-controlled study using acetaminophen as a side comparator. Arthritis Rheum 2007;56:555–67.
4. Towheed TE, Anastassiades T. Glucosamine therapy for osteoarthritis: an update. J Rheumatol 2007;34:1787–90.
5. Watterson JR, Esdaile JM. Viscosupplementation: therapeutic mechanisms and clinical potential in osteoarthritis of the knee. J Am Acad Orthop Surg 2000;8: 277–84.
6. Rutjes AW, Juni P, da Costa BR, et al. Viscosupplementation for osteoarthritis of the knee: a systematic review and meta-analysis. Ann Intern Med 2012;157:180–91.
7. Salk RS, Chang TJ, D'Costa WF, et al. Sodium hyaluronate in the treatment of osteoarthritis of the ankle: a controlled, randomized, double-blind pilot study. J Bone Joint Surg Am 2006;88:295–302.
8. Sun SF, Hsu CW, Sun HP, et al. The effect of three weekly intra-articular injections of hyaluronate on pain, function, and balance in patients with unilateral ankle arthritis. J Bone Joint Surg Am 2011;93:1720–6.
9. DeGroot H 3rd, Uzunishvili S, Weir R, et al. Intra-articular injection of hyaluronic acid is not superior to saline solution injection for ankle arthritis: a randomized, double-blind, placebo-controlled study. J Bone Joint Surg Am 2012;94:2–8.
10. Karatosun V, Unver B, Ozden A, et al. Intra-articular hyaluronic acid compared to exercise therapy in osteoarthritis of the ankle: a prospective randomized trial with long-term follow-up. Clin Exp Rheumatol 2008;26:288–94.
11. Boswell SG, Cole BJ, Sundman EA, et al. Platelet-rich plasma: a milieu of bioactive factors. Arthroscopy 2012;28:429–39.
12. Soomekh DJ. Current concepts for the use of platelet-rich plasma in the foot and ankle. Clin Podiatr Med Surg 2011;28:155–70.
13. Bibbo C, Hatfield PS. Platelet-rich plasma concentrate to augment bone fusion. Foot Ankle Clin 2010;15:641–9.
14. Jia X, Peters PG, Schon L. The use of platelet-rich plasma in the management of foot and ankle conditions. Oper Tech Sports Med 2011;19:177–84.
15. Steinert AF, Middleton KK, Araujo PH, et al. Platelet-rich plasma in orthopaedic surgery and sports medicine: pearls, pitfalls, and new trends in research. Oper Tech Orthop 2012;22:91–103.
16. Kon E, Mandelbaum B, Buda R, et al. Platelet-rich plasma intra-articular injection versus hyaluronic acid viscosupplementation as treatments for cartilage pathology: from early degeneration to osteoarthritis. Arthroscopy 2011;27:1490–501.

17. Kitaoka HB. Arthrodesis of the ankle: technique, complications, and salvage treatment. Instr Course Lect 1999;48:255–61.
18. Thomas RH, Daniels TR. Ankle arthritis. J Bone Joint Surg Am 2003;85:923–36.
19. Bjordal JM, Johnson MI, Lopes-Martins RA, et al. Short-term efficacy of physical interventions in osteoarthritic knee pain. A systematic review and meta-analysis of randomized placebo-controlled trials. BMC Musculoskelet Disord 2007;8:51.
20. Arroll B, Goodyear-Smith F. Corticosteroid injections for osteoarthritis of the knee: meta-analysis. BMJ 2004;328:869.
21. Ayral X. Injections in the treatment of osteoarthritis. Best Pract Res Clin Rheumatol 2001;15:609–26.
22. Creamer P. Intra-articular corticosteroid treatment in osteoarthritis. Curr Opin Rheumatol 1999;11:417–21.
23. Shih LY, Wu JJ, Lo WH. Changes in gait and maximum ankle torque in patients with ankle arthritis. Foot Ankle 1993;14:97–103.
24. Roos EM, Dahlberg L. Positive effects of moderate exercise on glycosaminoglycan content in knee cartilage. Arthritis Rheum 2005;52:3507–14.
25. Vlieland T, Pattison D. Non-drug therapies in early rheumatoid arthritis. Best Pract Res Clin Rheumatol 2009;23:103–16.
26. Anain JM Jr, Bojrab AR, Rhinehart FC. Conservative treatment for rheumatoid arthritis in the foot and ankle. Clin Podiatr Med Surg 2010;27:193–207.
27. Imboden J, Hellmann D, Stone J. Transcutaneous electrical nerve stimulation. Cur Rheumatol Diag Treat 2006;2:454.
28. Christie A, Jamtvedt G, Thuve Dahm K, et al. Effectiveness of nonpharmacological and nonsurgical interventions for patient with rheumatoid arthritis: an overview of systemic reviews. Phys Ther 2007;87:12.
29. Ayling J, Marks R. Efficacy of paraffin wax baths for rheumatoid arthritic hands. Physiotherapy 2000;86:190–201.
30. Robinson VI, Brosseau L, Casimiro LY, et al. Thermotherapy for treating rheumatoid arthritis. Cochrane Database Syst Rev 2002;(2):CD002826.
31. Brosseau L, Judd MG, Marchand S, et al. Transcutaneous electrical nerve stimulation (TENS) for the treatment of rheumatoid arthritis in the hand. Cochrane Database Syst Rev 2006;(1):CD004377.
32. Ottawa Panel. Ottawa panel evidence-based clinical practice guidelines for electrotherapy and thermotherapy interventions in the management of rheumatoid arthritis in adults. Phys Ther 2004;84:1016–43.
33. John S, Bongiovanni F. Brace management for ankle arthritis. Clin Podiatr Med Surg 2009;26:193–7.
34. Krause FG, Wing KJ, Younger AS. Neuromuscular issues in cavovarus foot. Foot Ankle Clin 2008;13:243–58.
35. Huang YC, Harbst K, Kotajarvi B, et al. Effects of ankle-foot orthoses on ankle and foot kinematics in patients with ankle osteoarthritis. Arch Phys Med Rehabil 2006;87:710–6.
36. Kitaoka HB, Crevoisier XM, Harbst K, et al. The effect of custom-made braces for the ankle and hindfoot on ankle and foot kinematics and ground reaction forces. Arch Phys Med Rehabil 2006;87:130–5.
37. Rao S, Ellis SJ, Deland JT, et al. Nonmedicinal therapy in the management of ankle arthritis. Curr Opin Rheumatol 2010;22:1–6.
38. Wu WL, Rosenbaum D, Su FC. The effects of rocker sole and SACH heel on kinematics in gait. Med Eng Phys 2004;26:639–46.
39. Kavlak Y, Uygur F, Korkmaz C, et al. Outcome of orthoses intervention in rheumatoid foot. Foot Ankle Int 2003;23(6):494–9.

40. Peltonen M, Lindroos AK, Torgerson JS. Musculoskeletal pain in the obese: a comparison with a general population and long-term changes after conventional and surgical obesity treatment. Pain 2003;104:549–57.
41. Wearing SC, Hennig EM, Byrne NM, et al. The biomechanics of restricted movement in adult obesity. Obes Rev 2006;7:13–24.
42. Aaboe J, Bliddal H, Messier SP, et al. Effects of an intensive weight loss program on knee joint loading in obese adults with knee osteoarthritis. Osteoarthr Cartil 2011;19:822–8.
43. Anandacoomarasamy A, Leibman S, Smith G, et al. Weight loss in obese people has structure-modifying effects on medial but not on lateral knee articular cartilage. Ann Rheum Dis 2012;71:26–32.
44. Frey C, Zamora J. The effects of obesity on orthopaedic foot and ankle pathology. Foot Ankle Int 2007;28:996–9.

Is There Any Value to Arthroscopic Debridement of Ankle Osteoarthritis and Impingement?

Phinit Phisitkul, MD*, Joshua N. Tennant, MD, MPH,
Annunziato Amendola, MD

KEYWORDS

- Ankle osteoarthritis • Arthroscopy • Treatment • Diagnosis • Debridement
- Impingement

KEY POINTS

- Evidence exists to support the use of arthroscopy in the diagnosis and treatment of ankle impingement, both soft tissue and osseous.
- Outcomes are less predictable in advanced ankle osteoarthritis with joint space narrowing.
- Alternative treatments of which arthroscopy is a component may also be a consideration in patients with more advanced ankle osteoarthritis.
- A meticulous debridement technique and early postoperative range-of-motion rehabilitation are important keys to success.

INTRODUCTION

Although Burman's 1931 cadaveric study stated that the ankle was not suitable for arthroscopy given the convexity of the talus, ankle arthroscopy has become a versatile technique and an increasingly popular tool in the diagnosis and treatment of a variety of ankle pathologies.[1] While some controversy exists regarding arthroscopic debridement of early ankle osteoarthritis and impingement, there is evidence to support benefit of the treatment. By allowing direct, minimally invasive visualization and manipulation of intra-articular structures, ankle arthroscopy offers an important surgical option for the properly selected patient. The authors strongly believe in the importance of proper indications and surgical techniques when treating patients by arthroscopic methods. This article provides an overview of the results from arthroscopic treatment of ankle arthritis and impingement with a review of the literature to date.

Department of Orthopaedics and Rehabilitation, University of Iowa Hospitals and Clinics, 200 Hawkins Drive, 0102X JPP, Iowa City, IA 52242-1088, USA
* Corresponding author.
E-mail address: phinit-phisitkul@uiowa.edu

Foot Ankle Clin N Am 18 (2013) 449–458
http://dx.doi.org/10.1016/j.fcl.2013.06.004
1083-7515/13/$ – see front matter Published by Elsevier Inc.

foot.theclinics.com

ANKLE OSTEOARTHRITIS AND ANTERIOR ANKLE IMPINGEMENT

Anterior impingement syndrome is a clinical diagnosis characterized by anterior ankle pain with painful limited dorsiflexion.[2,3] Anterior bone spur formation may be the result of repetitive microtrauma such as that endured by athletes likely by injury to the distal anterior cartilage rim just above the joint line as is seen in inversion injuries of the ankle.[3,4] Anterior impingement is more commonly described in the literature than posterior impingement, which may be associated with os trigonum syndrome or flexor hallucis longus tendinitis. The current literature on arthroscopic treatment of ankle impingement and osteoarthritis includes a large number of case series and reports, with some limited examples of higher-level evidence studies. Most of the studies support the use of arthroscopy in cases with impingement symptoms rather than in cases with advanced arthritic changes.

One recent systematic review of the literature on this topic has been performed. Glazebrook and colleagues[5] looked at the literature up to August 2008 for all indications for ankle arthroscopy, including treatment of impingement and osteoarthritis. Their review identified 1 level I study, 4 level II studies, 1 level III study, and 28 level IV case series. The summary findings presented graded recommendations for or against different indications, with impingement (anterior bone and soft tissue) receiving grade B (fair) evidence for intervention with arthroscopy, and ankle osteoarthritis grade C (poor) evidence against intervention. The 28 level IV case series, which included treatment of soft tissue impingement, bony impingement, and ankle osteoarthritis, showed a range of good or excellent patient outcomes in their results between 64% and 100%; most of the studies had more than 80% good outcomes. The authors of this systematic review found a general trend of improved postoperative outcomes in these case series in patients with soft tissue impingement compared with bony impingement, and increasingly poor results with increasing degree of ankle osteoarthritis.

Scranton and McDermott[6] compared open and arthroscopic debridement in a retrospective comparative (level III) study, finding that patients undergoing arthroscopic debridement had shorter hospital stays postoperatively. Although all patients showed some improvement after surgery, more severely degenerative ankles had a trend of longer recovery times. The investigators also developed a 1 to 4 grading system of anterior impingement based on severity and the location of osteophytes that is now commonly used in studies. A lower degree of spur formation correlated with a shorter time to return to full activity in the study.

Similar findings were concluded by van Dijk and colleagues[4] in a prospective cohort (level II) study comparing outcomes after arthroscopic debridement in patients with isolated anterior impingement with those with more advanced ankle osteoarthritis. Pain relief at 2 years after surgery was significantly better in the isolated anterior impingement group than in the osteoarthritis group. Patients without joint space narrowing had 90% good or excellent results, whereas patients with visible arthrosis on preoperative radiographs reported 50% good or excellent results. A longer preoperative time interval of symptoms was correlated with both increased grade of osteoarthritis and less postoperative satisfaction with the procedure.

Complete removal of impinging osteophytes may play an important role in the success of arthroscopic debridement. Takao and colleagues[7] found in a case-control (level III) study that three-dimensional preoperative computed tomography was helpful for identification and complete removal of anterior ankle osteophytes. This was demonstrated by an improvement in patients' postoperative American Orthopaedic Foot and Ankle Society (AOFAS) scores compared with the control group (only plain radiographs performed preoperatively), which was statistically significant at the latest follow-up in the study (average 24 months).

In a prospective cohort study of 26 patients (level III), Baums and colleagues[8] showed no statistically significant difference in clinical outcomes after 2 years between patients undergoing anterior soft tissue debridement (n = 12) compared with anterior bony debridement (n = 14), with 96% success overall (25 "very satisfied" patients and 1 "unsatisfied" patient). The 1 unsatisfied patient in the study had anterior bony impingement.

Kim and Ha[9] showed in a prospective cohort (level II) study that lateral ankle instability did not affect outcome postoperatively in 2 groups of patients who underwent arthroscopic anterolateral soft tissue debridement. Stability was defined as either increased anterior talar translation or talar tilt compared with the contralateral side as measured by stress radiographs with a Telos device (Acufex, Andover, MA). There were no significant differences between the 2 groups on subjective rating or ability to return to work, with overall 94% good or excellent results.

Han and colleagues[10] performed the only level I study to date in their randomized control trial of patients with previously arthroscopically confirmed syndesmosis instability with widening of more than 2 mm. Patients were randomized to syndesmotic fixation and arthroscopic anterolateral soft tissue debridement versus arthroscopic anterolateral soft tissue debridement alone, with equivalent improvement in AOFAS hindfoot score in both groups. The investigators' conclusion was that the anterolateral soft tissue was the primary source of pain, and that syndesmotic fixation is unnecessary if medial structures are stable.

Amendola and colleagues[11] reported that 24 of 29 patients undergoing an arthroscopic procedure for debridement of anterior bony or soft tissue ankle impingement reported benefitting from the procedure at a minimum of 2 years follow-up. In the same study, only 2 of 11 patients with ankle osteoarthritis or chondromalacia reported the same benefit. Ogilvie-Harris and colleagues[12] showed similar findings, with two-thirds of the 27 patient series showing some improvement after arthroscopy; there was a trend of greater improvement in milder preoperative cases of osteoarthritis.

The summary from these studies as well as several other level IV studies supported the general theme of the results of arthroscopic treatment in which success seemed to decline as the pathologies ranged from soft tissue impingement, osseous impingement, early osteoarthritis, to more advanced osteoarthritis (**Fig. 1**).[13–16]

OTHER TYPES OF ANKLE OSTEOARTHRITIS AND IMPINGEMENT

Although evidence is limited, arthroscopic debridement has shown benefits in the treatment of arthritic disorders that primarily involve synovium of the ankle joint including rheumatoid arthritis, localized pigmented villonodular synovitis, and hemophilic arthropathy (**Fig. 2**). Choi and colleagues[17] demonstrated 78% success of arthroscopic synovectomy in 18 consecutive patients with rheumatoid arthritis involving the ankle joint. The best clinical outcomes were achieved when the procedures were performed in early disease with minimal radiographic changes based on the Larsen grading system. A limited number of cases of arthroscopically treated localized pigmented villonodular synovitis have been reported with good success.[18–20] Arthroscopic synovectomy can be a definitive treatment when the extent of pathology is limited and without extra-articular involvement. Arthroscopy may help confirm the diagnosis and can be used as an adjunctive treatment with chemical or radioisotope synovectomy. In hemophilic arthropathy, arthroscopic synovectomy has shown promising results in the treatment of the ankle joint involvement.[21–24]

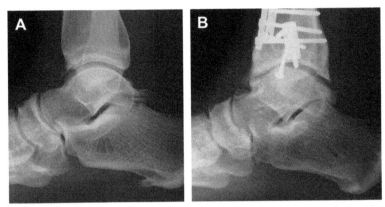

Fig. 1. Anterior ankle impingement. Lateral radiographs of patients with anterior ankle impingement are shown. Arthroscopic debridement has a good prognosis in patients with early arthritis and intact joint space (*A*) and a poor prognosis in patients with severe arthritis and joint space narrowing (*B*).

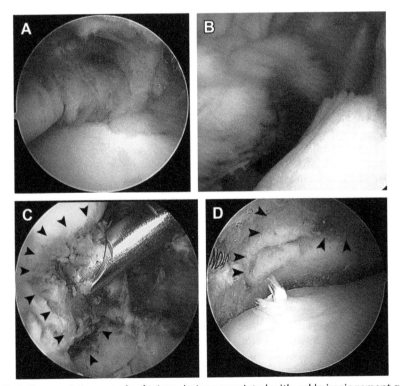

Fig. 2. Arthroscopic images of soft tissue lesions associated with ankle impingement symptoms. (*A*) Synovitis with soft tissue impingement. (*B*) Rheumatoid arthritis with synovial hyperplasia. (*C*) Pigmented villonodular synovitis (*arrowheads*). (*D*) Hemophilic arthropathy (*arrowheads* indicating hemosiderin laden synovium).

Benefits of this technique include improved functional outcomes, decreased frequency of hemarthrosis, and superior cost-effectiveness. Arthroscopic debridement has also been recommended in select cases of hemophilic arthropathy with advance ankle arthritis for the removal of loose cartilage and anterior osteophytes.[25]

Although posterior tibial osteophytes could be accessed and removed through posterior ankle arthroscopy, its role has not been established in the treatment of patients with ankle osteoarthritis. Ogut and colleagues[26] reported a 50% dissatisfaction rate after posterior ankle arthroscopic debridement in 8 patients with a diagnosis of osteoarthritis. These authors advised against the use of arthroscopic debridement in patients with generalized and posttraumatic arthritis.

ROLE OF DIAGNOSTIC ANKLE ARTHROSCOPY

Diagnosis of arthritic change by direct, minimally invasive visualization is afforded by ankle arthroscopy. Despite the emerging role of three-dimensional imaging studies, ankle arthroscopy is considered the gold standard in determining the true extent of cartilage damage in the ankle joint.[7,27,28] In 1979, Harrington[29] reported a case series on the use of arthroscopy in the evaluation of lateral ankle instability in 12 of 36 patients and confirmation of a diagnosis of medial ankle osteoarthritis. Takakura and colleagues[30] performed diagnostic arthroscopy to confirm the presence of intact cartilage on the lateral aspect of the tibiotalar joint before a corrective supramalleolar osteotomy in patients with ankle arthritis with varus deformity. Diagnostic arthroscopy also has a role in the prognostication of osteoarthritis development as a result of trauma, such as arthroscopy performed in conjunction with ankle fracture fixation.[31] The value of arthroscopy in the diagnosis of associated injuries that may lead to osteoarthritis has been repeatedly proposed in the evaluation of ankle syndesmotic disruption and deltoid ligament injury.[10,32–37]

ANKLE ARTHROSCOPY AS AN ADJUNCTIVE TREATMENT

Ankle arthroscopy has a limited role as a sole treatment of advanced ankle osteoarthritis. However, it has been commonly applied as an adjunctive treatment with ankle distraction arthroplasty.[38–41] Ankle distraction using an external fixator is indicated as an alternative to ankle arthrodesis in relatively young patients with advanced ankle osteoarthritis. Ankle arthroscopy is commonly performed before the application of external fixator in the same operative setting to remove inflamed synovium, unstable cartilage, loose bodies, fibrosis, and impinging osteophytes (**Fig. 3**). It has also been used to perform a microfracture on areas of eburnated bone.[42] The debridement of

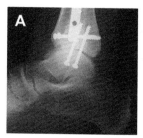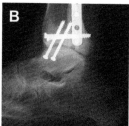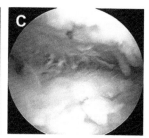

Fig. 3. Ankle arthroscopy and debridement together with ankle distraction. Preoperative and postoperative (*A, B*) lateral radiographs of a 24-year-old patient who underwent ankle arthroscopy and debridement together with ankle distraction are shown. Severe joint arthrofibrosis and loose cartilage flaps were arthroscopically debrided (*C*).

fibrosis and impinging osteophytes to obtain adequate dorsiflexion is critical to the success of the ankle distraction procedure.

In a level I study by Saltzman and colleagues,[41] ankle arthroscopy for the debridement of anterior osteophytes was used in all 36 patients undergoing ankle distraction. The investigators used the following methods to determine the adequacy of the debridement: (1) resection of the anterior tibial bone spur to the level of the anterior margin of the medial malleolus (2) visual assessment and removal of any anterior joint impingement, and (3) intraoperative inspection of true lateral fluoroscopic images. Two multicenter studies reported the use of arthroscopy in approximately two-thirds of the patients undergoing removal of fibrosis and osteophytes.[38,39] In contrast, Tellisi and colleagues performed ankle arthroscopy in only 4 of 25 patients who underwent ankle distraction.

Carpenter and colleagues[43] compared the results of ankle arthroscopy alone with combined ankle arthroscopy and hylan G-F 20 injections in 26 patients affected by at least grade II ankle osteoarthritis, according to the Kellgren-Lawrence scale. At a median follow-up of 13 months, the investigators found significant improvement in pain in both groups compared with the preoperative status. Those who received combined treatment had significantly more pain relief than arthroscopy alone. Although the invention of biological modalities may continue to enhance the emerging role of ankle arthroscopy, its present use cannot be recommended from the current evidence.

INDICATIONS

The indications of ankle arthroscopy for patients with ankle osteoarthritis are listed in **Box 1**. The patient should initially be adequately treated by nonsurgical methods for at least 3 to 6 months before proceeding to ankle arthroscopy. Radiographic evaluation should include weight-bearing anteroposterior, lateral, and Mortise views of the ankle. The Saltzman hindfoot alignment view is helpful for the evaluation of hindfoot deformity. A computed tomography scan is advisable for the preoperative mapping of size, shape, and number of osteophytes or loose bodies. Magnetic resonance imaging can be used to assist in the diagnosis of soft tissue lesions and cartilage damage especially for pigmented villonodular synovitis and hemophilic arthropathy. The patients should be counseled about the expectations and possible complications from arthroscopic treatment.

AUTHORS' PREFERRED TECHNIQUE

The patient is placed in the supine position with a thigh tourniquet. Ankle distraction is not required as most of the work is performed in the anterior aspect of the joint.

Box 1
Indications of ankle arthroscopy in ankle osteoarthritis

Early-stage ankle osteoarthritis with intact joint space

- Diagnostic arthroscopy and loose body removal
- Anterior ankle impingement
- Inflammatory arthropathy
- Pigmented villonodular synovitis
- Hemophilic arthropathy

Advanced-stage ankle osteoarthritis with joint space narrowing

- Ankle distraction

A 4-mm arthroscope is typically used with normal saline pump-assisted irrigation. The ankle joint can be insufflated with a 10 mL syringe and an 18-gauge needle. Standard anteromedial and anterolateral portals are marked on the skin at the level of the joint line. Each portal is established by making a skin incision followed by bluntly dissecting through soft tissue with a small hemostat to minimize the risk of injury to branches of the superficial peroneal nerve. As a certain degree of arthrofibrosis often coexists in an arthritic ankle, generous dilatation of the joint capsule is required for portal establishment. Occasionally, severe arthrofibrosis may prevent the placement of the instruments into the anterior joint capsule forcing the surgeon to start shaving extra-articularly (**Fig. 4**). Minimal debridement of the anterior capsule together with passive motion of the ankle joint facilitates the identification of the joint line in those severe cases. Loose bodies should be removed. Inflamed synovium is thoroughly debrided across the anterior recess, medial gutter, and lateral gutter of the ankle joint. Overzealous debridement of the soft tissue is avoided as the dorsalis pedis artery and the tarsal branches can be injured leading to a postoperative hematoma or a pseudoaneurysm.

Osteophytes are removed using a 4-mm acromioblast, a 4.5-mm full-radius shaver, or a narrow osteotome. The adequacy of anterior tibial debridement should be confirmed by the absence of impingement on passive maximum dorsiflexion with or without fluoroscopic guidance. Occasionally, an osteophyte or a cam lesion at the neck of the talus may cause impingement on full dorsiflexion. In this situation, we prefer to debride the junction between the talar dome and the talar neck to recreate a normal contour of the neck of talus under fluoroscopic guidance (**Fig. 5**). Medial gutter impingement can also be missed without a thorough evaluation. The arthroscope should be placed through the anterolateral portal and a shaver or a burr from the anteromedial portal. Osteophytes from the anterior aspect of the medial malleolus, the tip of the medial malleolus, and the medial aspect of the talar neck are identified and removed until impingement is absent.

The ankle is thoroughly examined to assess the extent of cartilage damage. Loose cartilaginous flaps are debrided to the stable rim. We do not recommend microfracture

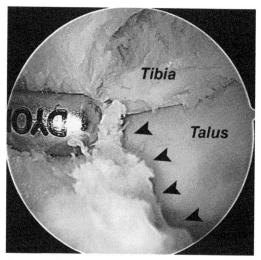

Fig. 4. Arthroscopic image with thickened anterior joint capsule (*arrow heads*) in an ankle with arthrofibrosis.

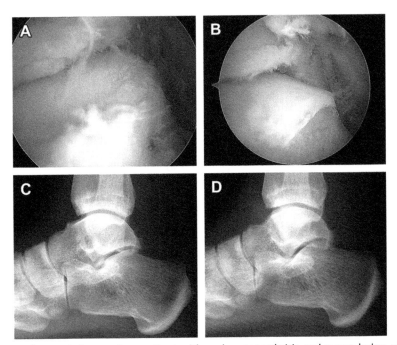

Fig. 5. Arthroscopic images in a patient with early osteoarthritis and a cam lesion at the talar neck reveal cartilage damage on both tibial and talar sides (A) and the status after arthroscopic debridement (B). Lateral radiographs of the same ankle demonstrate complete removal of anterior talar and tibial osteophytes (C, D).

treatment of eburnated bone except when the procedure is performed in conjunction with ankle distraction arthroplasty.

The patient is allowed to walk in a boot right away. Ankle range-of-motion exercise is crucial and must be initiated within a day or two after surgery to prevent equinus contracture. The exercise should be performed in a sitting position to relax the gastrocnemius muscles. A night splint is used for the first 6 weeks.

SUMMARY

Ankle arthroscopy can be valuable for the treatment of early-stage osteoarthritis with impingement symptoms from osseous or soft tissue lesions. It can also be used for joint evaluation and as an adjunctive treatment with other modalities. Meticulous surgical techniques and early postoperative motion are essential to achieve a successful outcome.

REFERENCES

1. Burman MS. Arthroscopy or the direct visualization of joints: an experimental cadaver study. J Bone Joint Surg 1931;13:695–9.
2. O'Donoghue DH. Impingement exostoses of the talus and tibia. J Bone Joint Surg Am 1957;39(4):835–52 [discussion: 852].
3. McMurray T. Footballer's ankle. J Bone Joint Surg Br 1950;32(1):68–9.
4. van Dijk CN, Tol JL, Verheyen CC. A prospective study of prognostic factors concerning the outcome of arthroscopic surgery for anterior ankle impingement. Am J Sports Med 1997;25(6):737–45.

5. Glazebrook MA, Ganapathy V, Bridge MA, et al. Evidence-based indications for ankle arthroscopy. Arthroscopy 2009;25(12):1478–90.

6. Scranton PE Jr, McDermott JE. Anterior tibiotalar spurs: a comparison of open versus arthroscopic debridement. Foot Ankle 1992;13(3):125–9.

7. Takao M, Uchio Y, Naito K, et al. Arthroscopic treatment for anterior impingement exostosis of the ankle: application of three-dimensional computed tomography. Foot Ankle Int 2004;25(2):59–62.

8. Baums MH, Kahl E, Schultz W, et al. Clinical outcome of the arthroscopic management of sports-related "anterior ankle pain": a prospective study. Knee Surg Sports Traumatol Arthrosc 2006;14(5):482–6.

9. Kim SH, Ha KI. Arthroscopic treatment for impingement of the anterolateral soft tissues of the ankle. J Bone Joint Surg Br 2000;82(7):1019–21.

10. Han SH, Lee JW, Kim S, et al. Chronic tibiofibular syndesmosis injury: the diagnostic efficiency of magnetic resonance imaging and comparative analysis of operative treatment. Foot Ankle Int 2007;28(3):336–42.

11. Amendola A, Petrik J, Webster-Bogaert S. Ankle arthroscopy: outcome in 79 consecutive patients. Arthroscopy 1996;12(5):565–73.

12. Ogilvie-Harris DJ, Sekyi-Otu A. Arthroscopic debridement for the osteoarthritic ankle. Arthroscopy 1995;11(4):433–6.

13. Hassouna H, Kumar S, Bendall S. Arthroscopic ankle debridement: 5-year survival analysis. Acta Orthop Belg 2007;73(6):737–40.

14. Loong TW, Mitra AK, Tan SK. Role of arthroscopy in ankle disorder–early experience. Ann Acad Med Singapore 1994;23(3):348–50.

15. Martin DF, Baker CL, Curl WW, et al. Operative ankle arthroscopy. Long-term followup. Am J Sports Med 1989;17(1):16–23 [discussion: 23].

16. Parisien JS, Vangsness T. Operative arthroscopy of the ankle. Three years' experience. Clin Orthop Relat Res 1985;(199):46–53.

17. Choi WJ, Choi GW, Lee JW. Arthroscopic synovectomy of the ankle in rheumatoid arthritis. Arthroscopy 2013;29(1):133–40.

18. Pavlica L, Nikolic D, Tadic J, et al. Pigmented villonodular synovitis–analysis of 50 patients. Vojnosanit Pregl 1997;54(3):209–16 [in Serbian].

19. Eisold S, Fritz T, Buhl K, et al. Pigmented villonodular synovitis. Case reports and review of the literature. Chirurg 1998;69(3):284–90 [in German].

20. Ottaviani S, Ayral X, Dougados M, et al. Pigmented villonodular synovitis: a retrospective single-center study of 122 cases and review of the literature. Semin Arthritis Rheum 2011;40(6):539–46.

21. Gilbert MS, Radomisli TE. Therapeutic options in the management of hemophilic synovitis. Clin Orthop Relat Res 1997;(343):88–92.

22. Patti JE, Mayo WE. Arthroscopic synovectomy for recurrent hemarthrosis of the ankle in hemophilia. Arthroscopy 1996;12(6):652–6.

23. Rodriguez-Merchan EC. Ankle surgery in haemophilia with special emphasis on arthroscopic debridement. Haemophilia 2008;14(5):913–9.

24. Tamurian RM, Spencer EE, Wojtys EM. The role of arthroscopic synovectomy in the management of hemarthrosis in hemophilia patients: financial perspectives. Arthroscopy 2002;18(7):789–94.

25. Pasta G, Forsyth A, Merchan CR, et al. Orthopaedic management of haemophilia arthropathy of the ankle. Haemophilia 2008;14(Suppl 3):170–6.

26. Ogut T, Ayhan E, Irgit K, et al. Endoscopic treatment of posterior ankle pain. Knee Surg Sports Traumatol Arthrosc 2011;19(8):1355–61.

27. Moon JS, Shim JC, Suh JS, et al. Radiographic predictability of cartilage damage in medial ankle osteoarthritis. Clin Orthop Relat Res 2010;468(8):2188–97.

28. Sugimoto K, Takakura Y, Okahashi K, et al. Chondral injuries of the ankle with recurrent lateral instability: an arthroscopic study. J Bone Joint Surg Am 2009; 91(1):99–106.

29. Harrington KD. Degenerative arthritis of the ankle secondary to long-standing lateral ligament instability. J Bone Joint Surg Am 1979;61(3):354–61.

30. Takakura Y, Tanaka Y, Kumai T, et al. Low tibial osteotomy for osteoarthritis of the ankle. Results of a new operation in 18 patients. J Bone Joint Surg Br 1995;77(1): 50–4.

31. Stufkens SA, Knupp M, Horisberger M, et al. Cartilage lesions and the development of osteoarthritis after internal fixation of ankle fractures: a prospective study. J Bone Joint Surg Am 2010;92(2):279–86.

32. Buchhorn T, Sabeti-Aschraf M, Dlaska CE, et al. Combined medial and lateral anatomic ligament reconstruction for chronic rotational instability of the ankle. Foot Ankle Int 2011;32(12):1122–6.

33. Lui TH, Ip K, Chow HT. Comparison of radiologic and arthroscopic diagnoses of distal tibiofibular syndesmosis disruption in acute ankle fracture. Arthroscopy 2005;21(11):1370.

34. McCollum GA, van den Bekerom MP, Kerkhoffs GM, et al. Syndesmosis and deltoid ligament injuries in the athlete. Knee Surg Sports Traumatol Arthrosc 2013; 21(6):1328–37.

35. Ogilvie-Harris DJ, Reed SC. Disruption of the ankle syndesmosis: diagnosis and treatment by arthroscopic surgery. Arthroscopy 1994;10(5):561–8.

36. Stufkens SA, van den Bekerom MP, Knupp M, et al. The diagnosis and treatment of deltoid ligament lesions in supination-external rotation ankle fractures: a review. Strategies Trauma Limb Reconstr 2012;7(2):73–85.

37. Takao M, Ochi M, Naito K, et al. Arthroscopic diagnosis of tibiofibular syndesmosis disruption. Arthroscopy 2001;17(8):836–43.

38. van Valburg AA, van Roermund PM, Marijnissen AC, et al. Joint distraction in treatment of osteoarthritis: a two-year follow-up of the ankle. Osteoarthritis Cartilage 1999;7(5):474–9.

39. Marijnissen AC, Van Roermund PM, Van Melkebeek J, et al. Clinical benefit of joint distraction in the treatment of severe osteoarthritis of the ankle: proof of concept in an open prospective study and in a randomized controlled study. Arthritis Rheum 2002;46(11):2893–902.

40. Chiodo CP, McGarvey W. Joint distraction for the treatment of ankle osteoarthritis. Foot Ankle Clin 2004;9(3):541–53, ix.

41. Saltzman CL, Hillis SL, Stolley MP, et al. Motion versus fixed distraction of the joint in the treatment of ankle osteoarthritis: a prospective randomized controlled trial. J Bone Joint Surg Am 2012;94(11):961–70.

42. Tellisi N, Fragomen AT, Kleinman D, et al. Joint preservation of the osteoarthritic ankle using distraction arthroplasty. Foot Ankle Int 2009;30(4):318–25.

43. Carpenter B, Motley T. The role of viscosupplementation in the ankle using hylan G-F 20. J Foot Ankle Surg 2008;47(5):377–84.

Ankle Joint Distraction Arthroplasty: Why and How?

Alexej Barg, MD[a,b], Annunziato Amendola, MD[c],
Douglas N. Beaman, MD[d], Charles L. Saltzman, MD[e,*]

KEYWORDS

- Ankle osteoarthritis • Joint-preserving treatment • Ankle joint distraction arthroplasty
- Motion distraction of the joint • Fixed distraction of the joint

KEY POINTS

- Ankle joint distraction has evolved as an alternative treatment option in patients with moderate or severe ankle osteoarthritis.
- Ideal candidates for ankle joint distraction are those patients with posttraumatic ankle osteoarthritis and are younger than 45 years.
- Two main fixation types can be used for ankle joint distraction: hinged distractor (ankle motion possible) or fixed distractor (no ankle motion possible).
- Postoperative pain relief is often incomplete. In patients with persisting pain and progressive ankle osteoarthritis, further therapeutic options like total ankle replacement or ankle arthrodesis can be easily performed.

INTRODUCTION

A growing number of patients are developing symptomatic ankle osteoarthritis from various causes.[1] Several clinical series (including the article by Barg and colleagues elsewhere in this issue) have shown that posttraumatic osteoarthritis is the most common cause in patients with end-stage ankle osteoarthritis.[2–4] Numerous treatment options have been described in the current literature for the different stages of ankle osteoarthritis and can be divided in joint-preserving and joint-nonpreserving procedures (**Fig. 1**). Patients with posttraumatic ankle osteoarthritis are usually younger

Disclosure: The authors have nothing to disclose.
[a] Orthopaedic Department, University Hospital of Basel, University of Basel, Spitalstrasse 21, Basel CH-4031, Switzerland; [b] Harold K. Dunn Orthopaedic Research Laboratory, University Orthopaedic Center, University of Utah, 590 Wakara Way, Salt Lake City, UT 84108, USA; [c] Department of Orthopaedics & Rehabilitation, University of Iowa Hospitals and Clinics, University of Iowa, 200 Hawkins Drive, Iowa City, IA 52242, USA; [d] Summin Orthopaedics LLP, 501 North Graham Street, Suite 250, Portland, OR 97227, USA; [e] University Orthopaedic Center, University of Utah, 590 Wakara Way, Salt Lake City, UT 84108, USA
* Corresponding author.
E-mail address: charles.saltzman@utah.edu

Foot Ankle Clin N Am 18 (2013) 459–470
http://dx.doi.org/10.1016/j.fcl.2013.06.005
1083-7515/13/$ – see front matter © 2013 Elsevier Inc. All rights reserved.

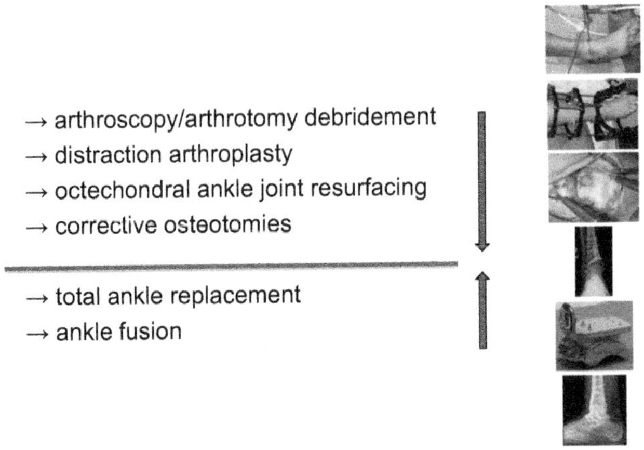

→ arthroscopy/arthrotomy debridement
→ distraction arthroplasty
→ octechondral ankle joint resurfacing
→ corrective osteotomies

_____

→ total ankle replacement
→ ankle fusion

Fig. 1. Stage-adapted treatment options of ankle osteoarthritis. Joint-preserving procedures: arthroscopic/open (eg, miniarthrotomy) debridement, distraction arthroplasty.

than patients with end-stage osteoarthritis of the hip or knee.[5] Ankle arthrodesis[6,7] and total ankle replacement[8,9] may relieve pain and provide good functional results, at least in the short-term. However, both surgical treatments have potential complications and long-term problems.[10–12] Therefore, in the younger and more active patient, joint-preserving procedures may be a better treatment option than total ankle replacement or ankle arthrodesis.

For select patients, distraction ankle arthroplasty may be a promising treatment approach for ankle osteoarthritis; however, there is still limited literature addressing its efficacy and clinical long-term results. Both treatment types of ankle osteoarthritis (with fixed and mobile distraction) have been described.[13–17]

In this article, the literature regarding the outcome after the distraction ankle arthroscopy is reviewed, the indications and contraindication for this procedure are listed, our surgical technique is described, and our preliminary results with this procedure are presented.

EFFICACY OF DISTRACTION ANKLE ARTHROPLASTY: LITERATURE REVIEW

Joint distraction with external fixation has evolved as an alternative treatment to joint-nonpreserving procedures like ankle arthrodesis or total ankle replacement.[18] The main idea behind this development was to address the intra-articular degenerative change and also to preserve the natural joint surfaces and ankle motion.[18] Another hypothesis as to how joint distraction should improve functional status of the ankle joint is that cartilage may self-repair when mechanical stress is removed, perhaps recapitulating ontogeny.[19,20] To our knowledge, the first reported joint distractions of the knee and elbow were performed in 1975[21] and of the ankle joint in 1978.[22] Aldegheri and colleagues[23] introduced the term arthrodiastasis to describe the distraction arthroplasty: *arthro* (joint), *dia* (through), and *tasis* (to stretch out).

Van Valburg and colleagues[16] treated 11 patients with posttraumatic ankle osteoarthritis with ankle joint distraction using the Ilizarov apparatus. Ankle distraction for 3 months resulted in substantial clinical improvement and pain relief. The range of movement was improved in 55% of all patients.[16] The same group presented the results of a prospective 2-year follow-up study including 17 consecutive patients.[17] The cause of osteoarthritis was different in this cohort; however, posttraumatic ankle osteoarthritis was the most common indication. Ilizarov external ring fixation was applied in all patients; in some of them, arthroscopic debridement was performed if needed. Ankle distraction was applied for 3 months, during which full weight-bearing was allowed as tolerated. Patients were followed for at least 1 year and in some cases, 4 to 8 years. In the entire cohort, more than two-thirds of the patients improved significantly as assessed by physical examination, functional ability questionnaires, and pain scale. The observed positive effects were progressive in the second postoperative year of follow-up. In 4 of 17 patients, distraction ankle arthroplasty did not result in substantial clinical or functional improvement. On average, ankle joint range of motion and radiographic joint space were preserved. In all cases, diminishing of subchondral sclerosis was observed.[17]

Van Roermund and Lafeber[15] presented a comprehensive review of this surgical technique. In general, these investigators described positive results after this procedure, including improved physical and functional results as well as pain relief and improved mobility. However, no statistical data were presented, patient recruitment was small and inefficient, and follow-up was inconsistent.[15]

Marijnissen and colleagues[24] performed a prospective trial along with a small randomized controlled trial of 17 patients comparing distraction ankle arthroplasty with ankle debridement. Substantial pain relief and improved functional scores were observed at between 1 and 3 years follow-up. However, these investigators did not find any statistically significant differences between the 2 small cohort groups.[25]

Ploegmakers and colleagues[25] addressed long-term benefit from joint distraction arthroplasty in 22 patients treated with Ilizarov joint distraction as a result of severe ankle osteoarthritis. The mean follow-up was 10 years. In 6 patients, ankle arthrodesis was performed because of increasing symptoms. In 16 patients, significant improvement in all clinical parameters, including patient satisfaction score, pain, and ankle osteoarthritis score, was observed.[25]

Rozbruch and Tellesi[26] used an Ilizarov external fixator in 25 patients with severe ankle osteoarthritis. At a minimum follow-up of 1 year, a significant improvement of American Orthopaedic Foot and Ankle Society (AOFAS) score from 55 points preoperatively to 75 postoperatively was observed. Furthermore, all components of the SF-36 survey improved substantially after surgery.[26]

Kanbe and colleagues[27] published a case report describing a 19-year-old female patient treated with ankle joint distraction as a result of severe chondrolysis. Motion distraction fixator was used for 4 weeks with ankle joint distraction of 5 mm. At 3-year follow-up, the patient was pain free, with normal clinical findings, including ankle and subtalar motion. The routine arthroscopy revealed fibrocartilage tissue lying between the talus and the tibia.[27]

Paley and colleagues[18] performed a thorough literature review and presented their surgical technique of how to apply distraction arthroplasty in patients with ankle osteoarthritis. Instead of the surgical technique presented by Dutch groups,[13,15–17,20–24,28] these investigators presented their Baltimore method; they preferred to build an ankle distractor with an anatomically located hinge, allowing range-of-motion exercises throughout distraction treatment. In total, 32 patients were treated by this surgical technique, in 18 of whom all follow-up data were completed. Positive outcomes were reported at the mean follow-up of 64 months (range, 24–157 months), with a mean AOFAS score of 71 points (range, 44–98 points).[18]

Tellisi and colleagues[29] presented a retrospective review of 25 patients who underwent distraction ankle arthroplasty. All patients had painful posttraumatic ankle osteoarthritis, with well-preserved ankle range of motion (at least 20°). A 2-ring fixator was used, with hinges placed along the axis of the ankle motion. The ankle was distracted approximately 5 mm. The frames were removed after 12 weeks after index surgery. No intraoperative or perioperative complications were observed in this study. The mean follow-up in this study was 30 months, ranging between 12 and 60 months. Most patients (91%) experienced substantial pain relief. The average AOFAS score significantly improved from 55 to 74. The motion of the tibiotalar joint was maintained in all patients. Two patients had undergone ankle arthrodesis because of progressive ankle osteoarthritis.[29]

Lamm and Gourdine-Shaw[30] presented their preliminary results in 3 patients treated with hinged ankle distraction, with a minimum of 1-year of follow-up. In all patients preoperative and postoperative T1-weighted and T2-weighted sagittal and coronal magnetic resonance imaging (MRI) scans were performed. The analysis of the MRI scans showed that the average postoperative subchondral bone thickness decreased by 0.5 mm and the average postoperative cartilage thickness increased by an average of 0.5 mm. The preoperatively observed subchondral bone cysts of the talus and tibia decreased in number and size.[30]

Ramanujam and colleagues[31] treated a 48-year-old man with posttraumatic tibiotalar and subtalar joint osteoarthritis as a result of a calcaneus fracture 2 years previously. Visualized transchondral lesions in the tibiotalar joint were debrided, addressed by using the microfracture technique, and treated using a collagen-glycosaminoglycan monolayer. A corrective arthrodesis was performed at the subtalar site. The prebuilt circular external fixator frame was positioned on the foot and lower extremity and removed 12 weeks postoperatively. At an average 8 months follow-up, the patient was satisfied and reported pain-free range of motion of the ankle. He was able to return to work and recreational activities without complaints.[31]

D'Angelantonio and Schick[32] presented a case report of ankle distraction using an external fixator with hinge articulation at the ankle joint in combination with joint resurfacing using an allograft. The external fixator was removed at 12 weeks. At follow-up 1 year postoperatively, this 61-year-old female patient was pain free and had no functional limitations.[32]

Van Meegeren and colleagues[33] treated 3 patients with hemophilic ankle arthropathy using joint distraction arthroplasty. Clinical and structural improvement was observed in this case series, resulting in high patient satisfaction.[33]

BIOCHEMICAL AND BIOMECHANICAL EFFECTS OF JOINT DISTRACTION IN OSTEOARTHRITIS

The biochemical and biomechanical basis behind the positive effects of joint distraction arthroplasty in ankles with osteoarthritis is complex. The ankle joint cartilage has different thickness and biomechanical properties than the knee and hip.[34] Therefore, the ankle cartilage may have a greater capacity for repair than that observed in the knee and hip.

Intema and colleagues[35] evaluated long-term changes in subchondral bone density in patients who underwent distraction ankle arthroplasty. Twenty-six patients with advanced posttraumatic ankle osteoarthritis were treated with joint distraction for 3 months using an Ilizarov frame. Dual-contrast computed tomography scans were performed before the treatment and at 1-year and 2-year follow-up, analyzing width of joint space and bone density. All patients in this study showed significant pain relief and functional improvement. Furthermore, decreases in subchondral bone density were observed postoperatively. These changes persisted during the entire follow-up period and may partially explain the clinical benefits of ankle joint distraction arthroplasty (**Fig. 2**).[35]

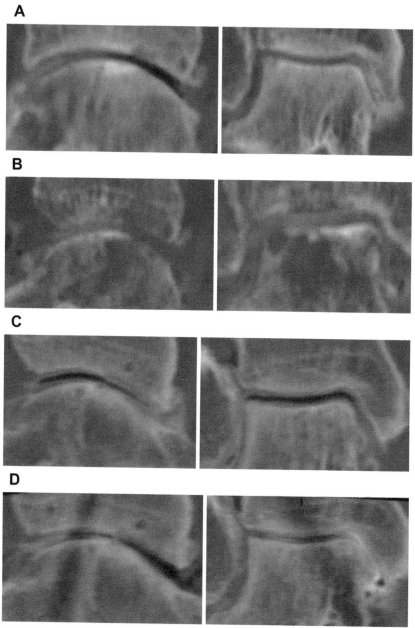

Fig. 2. Subchondral bone remodeling after ankle joint distraction arthroplasty. Severe bone disease at baseline (*A*) preoperatively and (*B*) directly after distraction, including cysts and sclerosis in the weight-bearing area. During the follow-up ([*C*] 1-year follow-up; [*D*] 2-year follow-up), a decrease of density in the sclerotic area was observed, whereas the cartilage layer seemed to increase.

Van Valburg and colleagues[36] used an animal model to address the effects of joint distraction on cartilage. Experimental osteoarthritis was induced in 13 beagle dogs by anterior cruciate ligament transection. All animals were divided into 3 groups: (1) with articulating joint distraction; (2) with nonarticulating joint distraction (blocked hinges); (3) no treatment. All histologic and biomechanical analyses were performed 25 weeks after the anterior cruciate ligament transection. Biochemical analysis showed that after joint distraction, the abnormal cartilage proteoglycan metabolism, characteristic for osteoarthritis, had changed to a level found in control uninjured joints. Furthermore, joint distraction reduced the mild degree of inflammation observed in osteoarthritic joints.[36]

Yanai and colleagues[37] investigated the effects of joint distraction and autologous bone-marrow–derived mesenchymal cell transplantation on repair of large full-thickness articular cartilage defects in an animal model. Thirty-three rabbits were included into this experimental study, consisting of 3 groups: (1) with and without joint distraction; (2) with joint distraction and collagen gel, and (3) with joint distraction and autologous bone-marrow–derived mesenchymal cell transplantation and collagen gel. The histologic score was significantly higher in the groups with autologous bone-marrow–derived mesenchymal cell transplantation collagen gel. The investigators concluded that joint distraction using a hinged fixator may reduce contact pressure on the regenerated area and results in the formation of a space required for cell proliferation and differentiation.[37] The investigators emphasized the use of a hinged fixator because the intermittent movement of the joint may provide the mechanical environment of hydrostatic pressure, resulting in appropriate proliferation of chondrocytes and production of lubrication for permeation of growth factors.[38,39] Similar findings were observed in an animal study performed by Nishino and colleagues.[40]

INDICATIONS AND CONTRAINDICATIONS FOR ANKLE JOINT DISTRACTION ARTHROPLASTY

Indications for ankle joint distraction arthroplasty are relatively congruent tibiotalar joint surface, pain, well-preserved ankle joint mobility, and moderate to severe osteoarthritis. Ideal candidates are those patients who have posttraumatic ankle osteoarthritis and are younger than 45 years.[41] Patients with partial avascular necrosis of the talus may be considered for this procedure.[18,30]

Contraindications for ankle joint distraction arthroplasty include, but are not limited to, the following: acute or chronic infection, osteomyelitis, arterial/venous insufficiency, neuropathy, Charcot arthropathy, psychosocial issues limiting the ability to maintain an external fixation device on the lower limb.

Relative contraindication for this procedure include uncontrolled diabetes, tobacco use, venous insufficiency with chronic venous dermatitis, chronic edema of the lower limb, severe ankle deformity, severe ankylosis of the ankle joint with no ankle motion, previous compartment syndrome with residual muscular-tendinous imbalance, and significant loss of bone stock.

Smith and colleagues[42] performed a comprehensive review of the current literature to provide a description of the level of evidence available to support ankle joint distraction arthroplasty for generally accepted indications. A total of 171 articles were reviewed and analyzed. Because of insufficient evidence-based literature, there is no clear support for the use of distraction ankle arthroplasty (**Table 1**). Because most of the published literature was literature reviews or expert opinion (level V), further high-quality studies are needed to highlight the efficacy of this surgical technique.[42]

Table 1
Summary of grade of recommendation for or against the current generally accepted indications for distraction ankle arthroplasty

Procedure	Grade of Recommendation
Posttraumatic osteoarthritis	I: for intervention
Degenerative joint disease	I: for intervention
Arthritis associated with ligamentous instability	I: for intervention
Chondrolysis	I: for intervention
Deformity associated with osteoarthritis	I: for intervention
Congenital abnormality	I: for intervention
Osteochondral defects	I: for intervention

Grades of recommendation for summaries or reviews of orthopedic surgical studies[43]:

A: Good evidence (level I studies with consistent findings) for or against recommending intervention.

B: Fair evidence (level II or III studies with consistent findings) for or against recommending intervention.

C: Poor quality evidence (level IV or IV with consistent findings) for or against recommending intervention.

I: there is insufficient or conflicting evidence not allowing a recommendation for or against intervention.

Data from Smith NC, Beaman D, Rozbruch SR, et al. Evidence-based indications for distraction ankle arthroplasty. Foot Ankle Int 2012;33(8):633.

SURGICAL TECHNIQUE

The procedure can be performed under general or regional anesthesia. The patient is placed supine on the operating table. A tourniquet is applied on the ipsilateral thigh, with pressure generally of 250 mm Hg. Before ankle joint distraction arthroplasty, we perform an anterior ankle arthroscopy using standard portals.[44,45] Arthroscopic ankle joint lavage is performed, with removal of any extra-articular anterior osseous osteophytes and intra-articular loose bodies using a 4.0-mm arthroscope without joint distraction. Plantar flexion of the ankle joint should be avoided, and the anterior capsule can be pulled over the joint, which may result in limitation of arthroscopic resection of anterior osteophytes. In patients in whom arthroscopic removal of anterior osteophytes is not possible because of the large extent of osteophytes, osteophytes should be removed using an anterior mini-incision through an extension of the arthroscopic portals. The adequacy of the anterior tibiotalar cheilectomy can be determined using the following parameters: (1) resection of the anterior tibial bone spur to the level of the anterior margin of the medial malleolus; (2) visual assessment and removal of any anterior tibiotalar joint impingement; and (3) intraoperative analysis of lateral fluoroscopic images through the dorsiflexion and plantarflexion of the ankle joint.[14]

The circumferential external fixator can be applied with (hinged distraction) and without (fixed distractor) motion. Motion frames have better outcomes.[14] The external fixator is applied in a standardized fashion, as planned preoperatively. First, the tibial frame is applied with the rings perpendicular to the longitudinal axis of the tibia. Second, the foot frame is placed in line with the foot. The tibial upper ring was secured with 2 5-mm half-pins and the lower ring was secured with 1 5-mm half-pin and a crossing 1.8-mm (thin) wire tensioned to 49.89 to 58.96 kg (110–130 lb). The foot frame was attached with a thin wire placed transversely across the talus, 2 crossing thin wires across the calcaneus, and 2 crossing thin wires across the metatarsals; all wired were tensioned to 31.75 to 40.82 (70 to 90 lb).

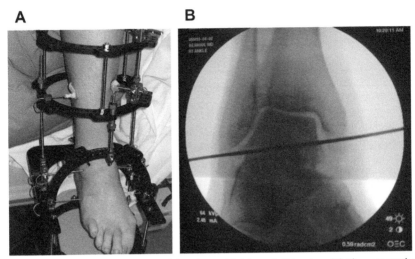

Fig. 3. (A) Clinical picture of external fixation with hinged distractor. (B) Fluroscopy shows the placement of Kirschner wire through the talus for distraction.

In cases with motion distraction (**Fig. 3**), distraction rods with hinges were used, with an unhinged posterior rod being detached during postoperative motion therapy. Universal hinges were placed at the level of the tips of the medial and lateral malleoli to approximate the mean location of the ankle joint axis.[46] In cases without motion (**Fig. 4**), distraction rods without hinges were used. In all cases, the ankle

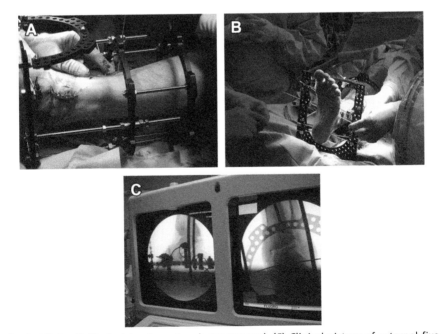

Fig. 4. (A) Small skin incision for osteophytes removal. (B) Clinical picture of external fixation with fixed distractor. (C) Fluoroscopy shows the correct placement of distractor and Kirschner wire through the talus.

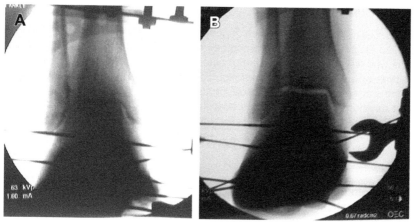

Fig. 5. Intraoperative ankle distraction. Anteroposterior radiographs of an ankle before (A) and after (B) thin-wire distraction.

joint was distracted about 5 mm, as assessed using intraoperative fluoroscopy (**Fig. 5**).

POSTOPERATIVE MANAGEMENT

Pin care is started 2 times daily until the pin sites are dry. They are not subsequently disturbed. Patients can take a shower and dab dry their pin sites. Full weight-bearing is allowed as tolerated (**Fig. 6**). Patients with motion distraction start with physiotherapy after the first week postoperatively. The external fixator is removed 3 months after the index surgery.

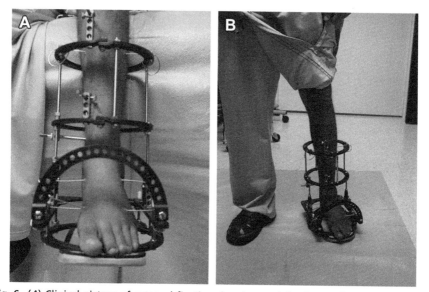

Fig. 6. (A) Clinical picture of external fixation showing no infection at the pin site. (B) Full weight-bearing with external fixator.

RESULTS OF TREATMENT

In 2012, Saltzman and colleagues[14] performed a level I prospective randomized controlled study comparing the outcomes for patients with advanced ankle osteoarthritis who were treated with anterior osteophyte removal and either (1) fixed ankle distraction or (2) hinged ankle distraction permitting joint motion. The follow-up was 24 months after frame removal in both groups. Subjects in both groups showed significant functional improvements as assessed using the Ankle Osteoarthritis Scale (AOS). Postoperatively, the motion-distraction group had significantly better AOS scores at different follow-up periods.

SUMMARY

Current literature reports and our results suggest that ankle joint distraction arthroplasty is a viable treatment option in younger patients with posttraumatic ankle osteoarthritis and well-preserved hindfoot motion. Pain relief is generally incomplete. In patients with persisting pain and progressive ankle osteoarthritis, further therapeutic options like total ankle replacement or ankle arthrodesis can be easily performed.

Further high-quality studies are required to address the efficacy of this procedure and to highlight long-term results in this patient cohort.

REFERENCES

1. Glazebrook M, Daniels T, Younger A, et al. Comparison of health-related quality of life between patients with end-stage ankle and hip arthrosis. J Bone Joint Surg Am 2008;90(3):499–505.
2. Saltzman CL, Salamon ML, Blanchard GM, et al. Epidemiology of ankle arthritis: report of a consecutive series of 639 patients from a tertiary orthopaedic center. Iowa Orthop J 2005;25:44–6.
3. Snedeker JG, Wirth SH, Espinosa N. Biomechanics of the normal and arthritic ankle joint. Foot Ankle Clin 2012;17(4):517–28.
4. Valderrabano V, Horisberger M, Russell I, et al. Etiology of ankle osteoarthritis. Clin Orthop Relat Res 2009;467(7):1800–6.
5. Brown TD, Johnston RC, Saltzman CL, et al. Posttraumatic osteoarthritis: a first estimate of incidence, prevalence, and burden of disease. J Orthop Trauma 2006;20(10):739–44.
6. Ahmad J, Raikin SM. Ankle arthrodesis: the simple and the complex. Foot Ankle Clin 2008;13(3):381–400, viii.
7. Raikin SM. Arthrodesis of the ankle: arthroscopic, mini-open, and open techniques. Foot Ankle Clin 2003;8(2):347–59.
8. Gougoulias N, Khanna A, Maffulli N. How successful are current ankle replacements?: a systematic review of the literature. Clin Orthop Relat Res 2010; 468(1):199–208.
9. Valderrabano V, Pagenstert GI, Muller AM, et al. Mobile- and fixed-bearing total ankle prostheses: is there really a difference? Foot Ankle Clin 2012;17(4):565–85.
10. Coester LM, Saltzman CL, Leupold J, et al. Long-term results following ankle arthrodesis for post-traumatic arthritis. J Bone Joint Surg Am 2001;83(2):219–28.
11. Glazebrook MA, Ganapathy V, Bridge MA, et al. Evidence-based indications for ankle arthroscopy. Arthroscopy 2009;25(12):1478–90.
12. Haddad SL, Coetzee JC, Estok R, et al. Intermediate and long-term outcomes of total ankle arthroplasty and ankle arthrodesis. A systematic review of the literature. J Bone Joint Surg Am 2007;89(9):1899–905.

13. Marijnissen AC, Vincken KL, Viergever MA, et al. Ankle images digital analysis (AIDA): digital measurement of joint space width and subchondral sclerosis on standard radiographs. Osteoarthritis Cartilage 2001;9(3):264–72.
14. Saltzman CL, Hillis SL, Stolley MP, et al. Motion versus fixed distraction of the joint in the treatment of ankle osteoarthritis: a prospective randomized controlled trial. J Bone Joint Surg Am 2012;94(11):961–70.
15. Van Roermund PM, Lafeber FP. Joint distraction as treatment for ankle osteoarthritis. Instr Course Lect 1999;48:249–54.
16. van Valburg AA, Van Roermund PM, Lammens J, et al. Can Ilizarov joint distraction delay the need for an arthrodesis of the ankle? A preliminary report. J Bone Joint Surg Br 1995;77(5):720–5.
17. van Valburg AA, Van Roermund PM, Marijnissen AC, et al. Joint distraction in treatment of osteoarthritis: a two-year follow-up of the ankle. Osteoarthritis Cartilage 1999;7(5):474–9.
18. Paley D, Lamm BM, Purohit RM, et al. Distraction arthroplasty of the ankle–how far can you stretch the indications? Foot Ankle Clin 2008;13(3):471–84, ix.
19. Sagray BA, Levitt BA, Zgonis T. Ankle arthrodiastasis and interpositional ankle exostectomy. Clin Podiatr Med Surg 2012;29(4):501–7.
20. Van Roermund PM, Marijnissen AC, Lafeber FP. Joint distraction as an alternative for the treatment of osteoarthritis. Foot Ankle Clin 2002;7(3):515–27.
21. Volkov MV, Oganesian OV. Restoration of function in the knee and elbow with a hinge-distractor apparatus. J Bone Joint Surg Am 1975;57(5):591–600.
22. Judet R, Judet T. The use of a hinge distraction apparatus after arthrolysis and arthroplasty (author's transl). Rev Chir Orthop Reparatrice Appar Mot 1978; 64(5):353–65 [in French].
23. Aldegheri R, Trivella G, Saleh M. Articulated distraction of the hip. Conservative surgery for arthritis in young patients. Clin Orthop Relat Res 1994;301: 94–101.
24. Marijnissen AC, Van Roermund PM, van Melkebeek J, et al. Clinical benefit of joint distraction in the treatment of severe osteoarthritis of the ankle: proof of concept in an open prospective study and in a randomized controlled study. Arthritis Rheum 2002;46(11):2893–902.
25. Ploegmakers JJ, Van Roermund PM, van Melkebeek J, et al. Prolonged clinical benefit from joint distraction in the treatment of ankle osteoarthritis. Osteoarthritis Cartilage 2005;13(7):582–8.
26. Trepman E, Lutter LD, Richardson EG, et al. Special report: highlights of the 23rd Annual Summer Meeting of the American Orthopaedic Foot And Ankle Society, Toronto, Ontario, Canada, July 13-15, 2007. Foot Ankle Int 2008;29(1):105–13.
27. Kanbe K, Hasegawa A, Takagishi K, et al. Arthroscopic findings of the joint distraction for the patient with chondrolysis of the ankle. Diagn Ther Endosc 1997;4(2):101–5.
28. Marijnissen AC, Van Roermund PM, van Melkebeek J, et al. Clinical benefit of joint distraction in the treatment of ankle osteoarthritis. Foot Ankle Clin 2003;8(2): 335–46.
29. Tellisi N, Fragomen AT, Kleinman D, et al. Joint preservation of the osteoarthritic ankle using distraction arthroplasty. Foot Ankle Int 2009;30(4):318–25.
30. Lamm BM, Gourdine-Shaw M. MRI evaluation of ankle distraction: a preliminary report. Clin Podiatr Med Surg 2009;26(2):185–91.
31. Ramanujam CL, Sagray B, Zgonis T. Subtalar joint arthrodesis, ankle arthrodiastasis, and talar dome resurfacing with the use of a collagen-glycosaminoglycan monolayer. Clin Podiatr Med Surg 2010;27(2):327–33.

32. D'Angelantonio AM, Schick FA. Ankle distraction arthroplasty combined with joint resurfacing for management of an osteochondral defect of the talus and concomitant osteoarthritis: a case report. J Foot Ankle Surg 2013;52(1):76–9.

33. van Meegeren ME, van Vulpen LF, Roosendaal G, et al. Joint distraction: a treatment to consider for haemophilic arthropathy. Haemophilia 2012;18(6):e418–20.

34. el Khoury GY, Alliman KJ, Lundberg HJ, et al. Cartilage thickness in cadaveric ankles: measurement with double-contrast multi-detector row CT arthrography versus MR imaging. Radiology 2004;233(3):768–73.

35. Intema F, Thomas TP, Anderson DD, et al. Subchondral bone remodeling is related to clinical improvement after joint distraction in the treatment of ankle osteoarthritis. Osteoarthritis Cartilage 2011;19(6):668–75.

36. van Valburg AA, Van Roermund PM, Marijnissen AC, et al. Joint distraction in treatment of osteoarthritis (II): effects on cartilage in a canine model. Osteoarthritis Cartilage 2000;8(1):1–8.

37. Yanai T, Ishii T, Chang F, et al. Repair of large full-thickness articular cartilage defects in the rabbit: the effects of joint distraction and autologous bone-marrow-derived mesenchymal cell transplantation. J Bone Joint Surg Br 2005; 87(5):721–9.

38. Tagil M, Aspenberg P. Cartilage induction by controlled mechanical stimulation in vivo. J Orthop Res 1999;17(2):200–4.

39. Mukherjee N, Saris DB, Schultz FM, et al. The enhancement of periosteal chondrogenesis in organ culture by dynamic fluid pressure. J Orthop Res 2001; 19(4):524–30.

40. Nishino T, Chang F, Ishii T, et al. Joint distraction and movement for repair of articular cartilage in a rabbit model with subsequent weight-bearing. J Bone Joint Surg Br 2010;92(7):1033–40.

41. Kluesner AJ, Wukich DK. Ankle arthrodiastasis. Clin Podiatr Med Surg 2009; 26(2):227–44.

42. Smith NC, Beaman D, Rozbruch SR, et al. Evidence-based indications for distraction ankle arthroplasty. Foot Ankle Int 2012;33(8):632–6.

43. Wright JG, Einhorn TA, Heckman JD. Grades of recommendation. J Bone Joint Surg Am 2005;87(9):1909–10.

44. Golano P, Vega J, Perez-Carro L, et al. Ankle anatomy for the arthroscopist. Part II: role of the ankle ligaments in soft tissue impingement. Foot Ankle Clin 2006; 11(2):275–96.

45. Golano P, Vega J, Perez-Carro L, et al. Ankle anatomy for the arthroscopist. Part I: the portals. Foot Ankle Clin 2006;11(2):253–73.

46. Bottlang M, Marsh JL, Brown TD. Articulated external fixation of the ankle: minimizing motion resistance by accurate axis alignment. J Biomech 1999;32(1): 63–70.

Management of Varus Ankle Osteoarthritis with Joint-Preserving Osteotomy

Mark S. Myerson, MD*, Jacob R. Zide, MD

KEYWORDS

- Osteotomy • Varus ankle arthritis • Tibiotalar joint

KEY POINTS

- The use of osteotomy in the treatment of varus ankle arthritis may delay or obviate the need for an ankle arthroplasty or arthrodesis.
- Deciding whether to perform an opening or closing wedge supramalleolar osteotomy is important to optimize surgical outcomes.
- The plafond-plasty is an osteotomy that can be helpful in the correction of intra-articular deformities.

The goal of osteotomy in the treatment of varus ankle arthritis is to shift the forces imparted to the ankle to a portion of the joint that is not involved in the degenerative process.[1–4] The redistribution of loads and stresses seen by the tibiotalar joint can be approached either above or below the ankle with an osteotomy of the tibia or calcaneus. Evaluation of the deformity as being subtalar, supramalleolar, or a combination allows the surgeon to best address the increased joint stresses, thereby reducing the risk of failure of the osteotomy.

Choosing the appropriate type of osteotomy for treatment of the deformity can optimize outcomes. The major advantage of the tibial opening wedge osteotomy is in the avoidance of leg shortening, but delayed union or nonunion may occur. Although leg length change may not seem significant if only 1 cm of shortening is performed with a wedge resection osteotomy, it must be kept in mind that the limb is already short from the deformity. Put another way, a deformity treated with an opening wedge that requires a 1-cm graft has a height differential of 2 cm compared with the same deformity treated instead with a closing wedge.[5] If there are skin-related problems (previous incisions with scar formation or prior infection) or if there is potential for vascular compromise, a closing wedge must be performed. Although the closing wedge

Institute for Foot and Ankle Reconstruction, Mercy Medical Center, 301 St. Paul Place, Baltimore, MD 21202, USA
* Corresponding author.
E-mail address: mark4feet@aol.com

Foot Ankle Clin N Am 18 (2013) 471–480
http://dx.doi.org/10.1016/j.fcl.2013.06.006
1083-7515/13/$ – see front matter © 2013 Elsevier Inc. All rights reserved.

foot.theclinics.com

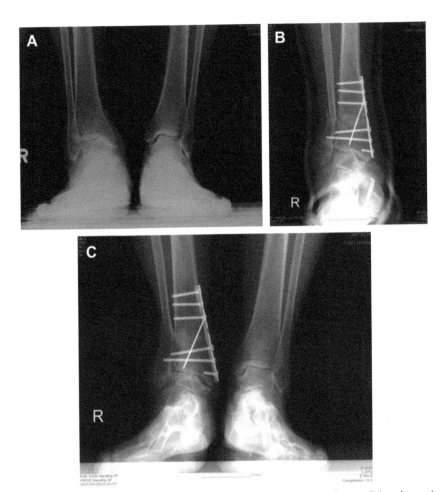

Fig. 1. (*A*) This patient was treated for varus ankle osteoarthritis with a traditional opening wedge supramalleolar osteotomy. Note the location of the osteotomy approximately 5 cm proximal to the articular surface. (*B*) Immediate postoperative radiographs. (*C*) Follow-up radiographs 2 years postoperatively. The orientation of this osteotomy is not able to accurately correct the varus ankle deformity. In the preoperative image, note the medialization of the talus and the flattening of the medial malleolus. This pattern is typical of medial compartment arthritis with or without varus ankle deformity. The postoperative image shows the slight lateral shift of the talus relative to the longitudinal axis of the tibia. This lateralization is beneficial because there is increased load on the lateral articular surface, but the center of the talus is no longer congruent with the center of the tibia. (*Courtesy of* Dr Woo Chun Lee, Seoul, South Korea.)

osteotomy results in leg shortening, it remains an attractive option because it is generally easier than the opening wedge procedure, particularly if this includes the fibula and the tibia.

For the correction of a varus deformity, we generally use either a medial opening wedge osteotomy or a lateral closing wedge osteotomy. The medial opening wedge osteotomy is performed through an anteromedial and a small lateral incision (for the fibular osteotomy). Which bone cut is made first is a matter of preference, but leaving

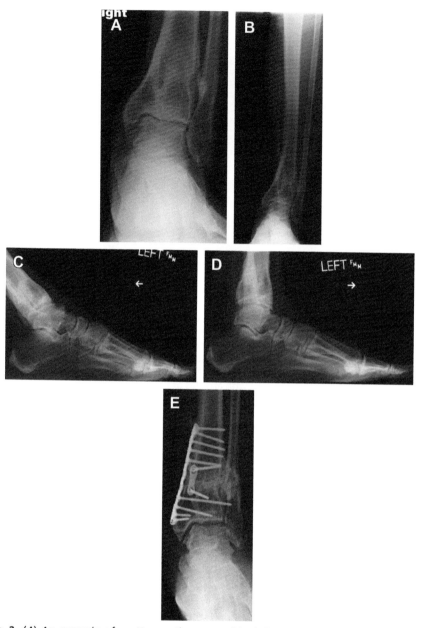

Fig. 2. (*A*) An example of posttraumatic varus ankle deformity treated with an opening wedge osteotomy. (*B*) Long leg radiograph obtained to evaluate the overall alignment of the limb. (*C, D*) Flexion and extension lateral views of the ankle are obtained to ascertain the true amount of motion coming from the ankle joint and can be used to evaluate for any sagittal plane deformity. The *arrows* in C and D indicate maximum plantarflexion and dorsiflexion of the ankle respectively. (*E*) An opening wedge medial osteotomy has been performed 4-cm proximal to the articular surface with excellent correction of ankle alignment. This is a good example of a typical posttraumatic deformity. Note the position of the center of rotation of angulation (CORA) here. This is the prototypical indication for the medial opening wedge distal tibia osteotomy, performed at the level of the CORA without concern for creating a secondary translational deformity. Note also the inclusion of the long leg view, which is very important in the context of this type of deformity, particularly because the patient has slight tibia vara in addition to the distal deformity. Flexion and extension views are an important consideration in planning treatment.

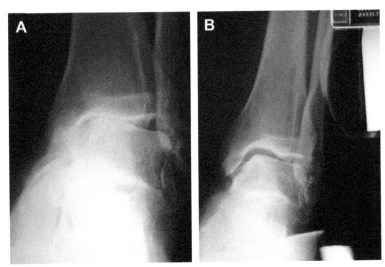

Fig. 3. (*A, B*) The evaluation of any varus ankle deformity should begin with stress images. Here in this 42-year-old man who presented with chronic ankle instability there is typical varus deformity associated with an erosion of the distal medial tibial plafond. This becomes more evident with the stress view where the indentation of the distal tibia is more noticeable. The ankle was reducible although it required considerable force to do so. Patients with chronic ankle instability often present with arthritis of the medial compartment of the ankle associated with an erosion of the distal medial tibia and a dysplastic medial malleolus.

the fibula intact provides some stability while the tibial cut is completed. When the deformity is minimal, then a greenstick cut of the tibia can be made with the hope that a fibular osteotomy may not need to be performed. A greenstick osteotomy markedly increases the stability of the cut, and the tibia can be opened with a lamina spreader to the desired amount of correction. If there is a concern that the lateral cortex will break, or if the planned opening wedge is too great to avoid making a complete cut, we apply a two- or three-hole plate to the lateral aspect of the distal tibia at the level where the osteotomy exits. This technique creates a hinge point for opening of the osteotomy, prevents overcorrection, and maintains tension on the lateral side of the cut. The plate should be applied just before the osteotomy cut exits the lateral tibial cortex.

The opening wedge osteotomy is performed 4 cm proximal to the medial malleolar tip in metaphyseal bone. Locating the cut in the metaphysis rather than another arbitrary location on the tibia provides a broad surface with good blood supply for healing of the graft. After the skin incision is made, periosteal stripping is kept to a minimum such that only an amount sufficient to complete the osteotomy is performed. Secure fixation is requisite and we apply the selected plate to the surface of the tibia to find the best location for making the osteotomy. Using the plate to mark the exact height of the cut ensures that sufficient space is maintained to obtain fixation with three screws distally. The bone cut is made perpendicular to the tibia with a broad oscillating saw, and when possible, the lateral cortex and periosteal sleeve are preserved to act as a fulcrum for the opening wedge and to enhance stability. If nothing more than uniplanar correction is required then this greenstick type of cut or a small plate over the lateral tibia is useful to prevent overcorrection. If biplanar deformity is present, or if translation and rotation are also necessary, then the opposite cortex must be cut to allow the distal segment to move. A fibular wedge osteotomy is generally performed

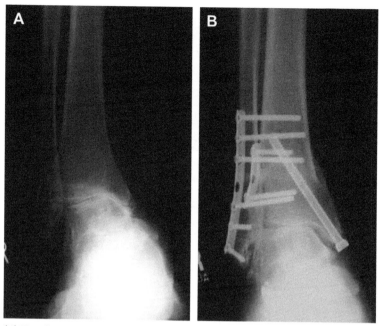

Fig. 4. (*A*) Here is a good example of varus ankle arthritis, with an oblique medial malleolus, medial distal intra-articular tibial erosion, medial translation of the talus under the tibia, and varus deformity of the hindfoot. (*B*) After lateral closing wedge osteotomy, the alignment of the plafond is much improved but the deformity has recurred because of persistence of the intra-articular deformity. Although a lateral closing wedge osteotomy may have a role in treating varus ankle osteoarthritis, it is limited to very specific types of deformity where the CORA is easily located in the distal tibia and the patient can tolerate the loss of 1 cm of limb length. In this 58-year-old patient, the deformity was the result of chronic ankle instability and not primary varus ankle osteoarthritis. Although the alignment of the ankle is much improved and the load is shifted to the lateral plafond, the deformity has recurred because of the chronic depression in the distal medial tibia, because the talus has a tendency to "drop back" into this position.

with the lateral incision at the same level as that for the tibial osteotomy, although this location is not critical.

After the osteotomy has been performed, a lamina spreader is inserted to gradually distract the osteotomy so that the ankle comes to rest in a neutral to slightly overcorrected position.[6–8] Ankle alignment is verified fluoroscopically. We prefer to use a structural femoral head allograft to fill the defect. The structural bone graft provides immediate mechanical support, with little likelihood of collapse even after resorption, which occurs during revascularization. Some structural integrity remains during the process of bone graft incorporation to allow the graft to withstand loads. After the deformity has been corrected, the graft is shaped and inserted and the osteotomy is provisionally fixed with K-wires. Fluoroscopy is used to check final alignment and the plate is affixed to the tibia with at least three screws proximal and distal to the cut (**Figs. 1** and **2**).

There are circumstances where the preservation of limb length is neither necessary nor desirable. For these patients, a closing wedge lateral osteotomy of the fibula and tibia is performed. The medial closing wedge is performed through a single lateral incision for the tibia and the fibula. A small separate incision is created medially to apply a

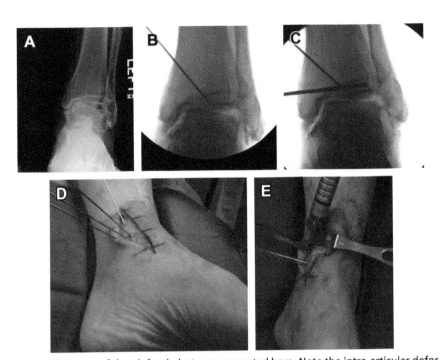

Fig. 5. (*A*) The steps of the plafond plasty are presented here. Note the intra-articular deformity with depression of the medial tibial plafond. (*B*) After a medial incision has been created over the tibia, a guide pin is inserted with the tip positioned at the apex of the intra-articular deformity. (*C*) Two K-wires have been inserted just proximal to the tibial plafond to prevent the saw from entering the joint, and to serve as a buttress to propagation of the osteotomy into the joint during the actual correction of the deformity. (*D–F*) Intraoperative photographs demonstrating position of the guide pins and saw. (*G*) The osteotomy is created with the saw aligned perpendicular to the coronal axis of the tibia. (*H, I*) Clinical and radiographic images showing displacement of the osteotomy with a lamina spreader for correction of the deformity. Note in the radiograph that although the transverse guide pins have bent, there is no propagation of the osteotomy into the plafond. (*J*) Final radiograph demonstrating correction of intra-articular depression and stabilization of the osteotomy with multiple screws. This is a good case for the plafond-plasty. There is not a considerable amount of deformity; however, there is an intra-articular divot in the distal medial tibia, and a standard supramalleolar osteotomy would not work here. Note the build up of bone around the medial malleolus. One has to consider debridement of these osteophytes. Although they do not preclude the sequence of the osteotomy steps, there is residual contracture around the medial malleolus, which may cause subsequent symptoms.

small plate to the tibia for prevention of overcorrection. The osteotomy can be tensioned against the fixed fulcrum medially with this technique.

As in the opening wedge osteotomy, the location of the osteotomy is within the metaphysis. The wedge resection can be marked by placing a lateral to medial K-wire perpendicular to the axis of the proximal tibia to mark the proximal extent of the planned cut. A second K-wire is placed distal to the first and parallel to the ankle joint surface such that the tips of the wires converge. These wires are placed with fluoroscopic guidance. A large oscillating saw is then used to remove the bony wedge marked by the wires. After a wedge has also been removed from the fibula, the tibial osteotomy is compressed and fixed with a plate.

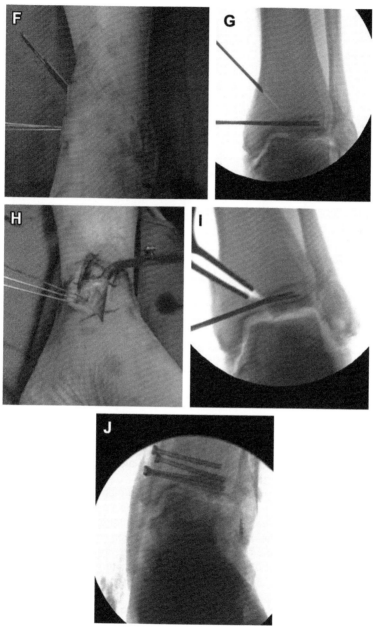

Fig. 5. (*continued*)

Fig. 3 shows an example of chronic lateral ankle instability, associated with a varus distal tibia. Previously, a lateral closing wedge osteotomy would have been used for correction of this type of deformity, but over the years, we have recognized that a defect of the medial distal tibia persists, and a recurrence of the varus of the ankle is likely. Although symptoms are markedly improved and stability is corrected with a

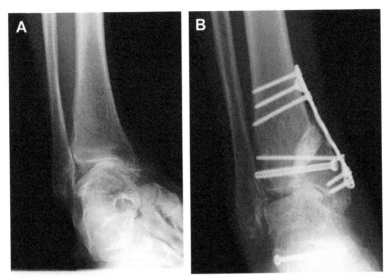

Fig. 6. (A) Severe varus ankle deformity with intra-articular erosion of the tibial plafond. (B) A plafond-plasty procedure was selected here as a staged osteotomy, knowing that a further subsequent procedure would likely be performed. The procedure was performed in the standard manner as outlined previously. Note the use of the distal screw in the tibia, required because the osteotomy opened up at the level of the joint surface and the screw closed this down. The choice of the plafond-plasty here is reasonable, albeit improbable that it alone would correct the deformity. A peroneus longus to brevis transfer in addition to ankle ligament reconstruction and an osteotomy of the first metatarsal was performed at the time of the plafond plasty osteotomy. This procedure had been planned intentionally as a staged correction before ankle replacement, which was performed successfully 6 months later.

standard supramalleolar osteotomy, these intra-articular deformities require a different approach, as discussed next.

In the past, the senior author (MSM) has attempted many different types of procedures to avoid an ankle arthrodesis or arthroplasty in the management of chronic ankle instability associated with varus hindfoot and a varus intra-articular deformity of the ankle. These included a lateral ligament reconstruction, peroneal tendon repair or transfer of the longus to the brevis, calcaneal osteotomy, and lateral opening or medial closing wedge osteotomies of the tibia and fibula. Although many of these procedures corrected one component of the problem, deformity frequently persisted or recurred because of the intra-articular component of the deformity. With chronic varus instability, there is an erosion of the medial distal tibia, and the talus falls into this defect resulting in ankle varus. Added to this, the medial malleolus begins to erode, and instead of a vertically orientated malleolus, it is medially inclined. Both of these anatomic abnormalities add to the likelihood of recurrent deformity. To correct this specific deformity we frequently use a modified intra-articular osteotomy, called the plafond-plasty for correction of this deformity (**Fig. 4**).

The plafond plasty osteotomy is performed in conjunction with additional hindfoot alignment and stabilization of the ankle as required. The medial distal tibia is exposed, and a guide pin is inserted to mark the plane of the osteotomy. The position of the guide pin is checked fluoroscopically. The pin should terminate at the level of the intra-articular defect of the tibia. Two or three additional guide pins are then inserted immediately above the ankle joint to function as a buttress and prevent the saw cut from entering the joint. A saw is used to perform the osteotomy along the plane of the guide pin, stopping immediately above the joint line. The osteotomy is then gradually opened with a broad osteotome, levering the distal tibia open. The joint is protected from extension of the osteotomy to the articular surface by the periarticular

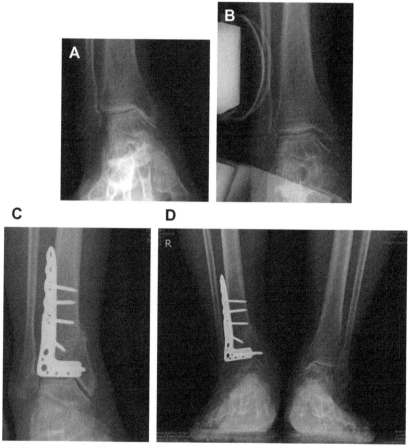

Fig. 7. (*A, B*) Varus ankle osteoarthritis with medial intra-articular erosion of the tibial plafond and flattening of the medial malleolus. (*C, D*) The deformity was corrected in this patient with a distal oblique osteotomy that exits just at the lateral corner of the joint. This is a variation of the plafond-plasty, where the osteotomy exits at the level of the plafond, but further laterally and obviously is not intra-articular. The advantage of this type of osteotomy is that it is not intra-articular. Note how well the medial malleolus orientation has been restored from an oblique to a more vertical position. The orientation of this osteotomy makes far more sense than a standard opening wedge supramalleolar osteotomy performed 4-cm proximal to the joint for management of varus ankle osteoarthritis. In our opinion the only indication for the latter procedure is for correction of congenital or traumatic deformity where a true CORA for the deformity exists in the metaphysis. (*Courtesy of Dr Woo Chun Lee, Seoul, South Korea.*)

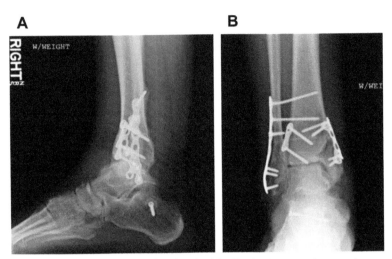

Fig. 8. (*A*, *B*) This patient was treated with a double distal osteotomy to correct varus of the distal tibia that was also associated with a varus intra-articular deformity. A closing wedge lateral osteotomy through the fibula and tibia was performed in a standard manner, and was then supplemented with a medial plafond-plasty procedure.

guide pins, which were inserted before the osteotomy. Cancellous bone graft is then used to fill the osteotomy, which is fixed with a plate (**Figs. 5–8**).

REFERENCES

1. Tarr RR, Resnick CT, Wagner KS, et al. Changes in tibiotalar joint contact areas following experimentally induced tibial angular deformities. Clin Orthop Relat Res 1985;199:72–80.
2. Ting AJ, Tarr RR, Sarmiento A, et al. The role of subtalar motion and ankle contact pressure changes from angular deformities of the tibia. Foot Ankle 1987;7(5): 290–9.
3. Knupp M, Stufkens SA, van Bergen CJ, et al. Effect of supramalleolar varus and valgus deformities on the tibiotalar joint: a cadaveric study. Foot Ankle Int 2011; 32(6):609–15.
4. Stufkens SA, van Bergen CJ, Blankevoort L, et al. The role of the fibula in varus and valgus deformity of the tibia. J Bone Joint Surg Br 2011;93:1232–9.
5. Canale ST, Harper MC. Biotrigonometric analysis and practical applications of osteotomies of tibia in children. Instr Course Lect 1981;30:85–101.
6. Lee W, Moon J, Lee K, et al. Indications for supramalleolar osteotomy in patients with ankle osteoarthritis and varus deformity. J Bone Joint Surg Am 2011;93: 1243–8.
7. Takakura Y, Tanaka Y, Kumai T, et al. Low tibial osteotomy for osteoarthritis of the ankle: results of a new operation in 18 patients. J Bone Joint Surg Br 1995;77: 50–4.
8. Knupp M, Hintermann B. Treatment of asymmetric arthritis of the ankle joint with suprmalleolar osteotomies. Foot Ankle Int 2012;33(3):250–2.

Joint-Preserving Surgery of Valgus Ankle Osteoarthritis

Victor Valderrabano, MD, PhD[a],*, Jochen Paul, MD[b],
Horisberger Monika, MD[b], Geert I. Pagenstert, MD[b],
Heath B. Henninger, PhD[c], Alexej Barg, MD[b,c]

KEYWORDS

- Valgus ankle osteoarthritis • Supramalleolar osteotomy
- Lateral lengthening calcaneal osteotomy • Medial displacement calcaneal osteotomy
- Cotton osteotomy

KEY POINTS

- The most common cause of ankle osteoarthritis is posttraumatic, often resulting in a concomitant valgus or varus deformity of the hindfoot.
- There are 2 main etiologic and morphologic groups of asymmetric valgus ankle osteoarthritis: primary form and posttraumatic form.
- In patients with valgus hindfoot deformity the lateralized mechanical lower leg axis leads to overload of the lateral compartment of the tibiotalar joint.
- Diagnosis of valgus ankle osteoarthritis is based on careful clinical assessment and radiographic imaging including weight-bearing radiographs of the foot and ankle.
- Before considering joint-preserving surgery in patients with valgus osteoarthritic ankle all contraindications should be excluded.
- The aim of joint-preserving surgery is to realign the hindfoot and to normalize the heel contact point. Overall, in the current literature promising short-term and mid-term results have been observed in patients who underwent realignment surgery due to valgus hindfoot deformity.

INTRODUCTION

Osteoarthritis (OA) is a growing problem in health care worldwide. Approximately 1% of the adult population suffers from painful end-stage ankle OA,[1] but ankle OA is

The authors have nothing to disclose.
[a] Orthopaedic Department, Osteoarthritis Research Center Basel, University Hospital of Basel, University of Basel, Spitalstrasse 21, Basel 4031, Switzerland; [b] Orthopaedic Department, University Hospital of Basel, University of Basel, Spitalstrasse 21, Basel CH-4031, Switzerland; [c] Department of Orthopaedics, Harold K. Dunn Orthopaedic Research Laboratory, University Orthopaedic Center, University of Utah, 590 Wakara Way, Salt Lake City, UT 84108, USA
* Corresponding author.
E-mail address: victor.valderrabano@usb.ch

significantly less common than in the knee or hip. However, the clinical importance of ankle OA should not be underestimated. Glazebrook and colleagues[1] have demonstrated that patients with end-stage ankle OA have mental and physical disability comparable with that of patients with end-stage hip OA.

The most common cause of ankle OA is posttraumatic, with around 80% of all incidences, followed by primary and secondary ankle OA.[2–4] The most common reason for developing posttraumatic ankle OA is a fracture of lower leg, but patients with repetitive ligamentous lesions and chronic ankle instability may also develop degenerative changes of the tibiotalar joint.[5] Patients with posttraumatic ankle OA typically present with asymmetric involvement of the tibiotalar joint, resulting in valgus or varus deformity of the ankle and hindfoot.[6] Without appropriate treatment, patients with asymmetric ankle OA typically develop full end-stage ankle OA in the mid or long term.[7,8]

Ankles with pathologic valgus deformities suffer from a lateral joint overload with subsequent lateral tibiotalar joint degeneration, which causes further lateral load shift (vicious circle).[7,9,10] In most cases the patients are younger than 50 years. More than half of the tibiotalar joint is typically preserved, so that joint-sacrificing procedures such as total ankle replacement or ankle arthrodesis may be not the most appropriate treatment options. In these cases patients may benefit from joint-preserving realignment surgery to unload the degenerated lateral area and normalize joint biomechanics. Short-term and mid-term results following realignment surgery are promising, with substantial postoperative pain relief and functional improvement that is reflected in high patient satisfaction.[8,11–13]

This article describes the authors' algorithm for the treatment of patients with asymmetric valgus ankle OA.

ETIOLOGY OF ASYMMETRIC VALGUS ANKLE OSTEOARTHRITIS

The etiology of asymmetric arthritic valgus ankles can be divided into 2 main etiologic and morphologic groups (**Table 1**).[14] The primary form of asymmetric valgus ankle OA is characterized by severe deformity of the pes planovalgus, with insufficiency of the medial ligaments and end-stage tibial tendon dysfunction (Grade IV using the Myerson classification).[14–19] Talocalcaneal and/or calcaneonavicular coalition may also be associated with asymmetric valgus ankle OA.[20] The second important etiologic category of asymmetric valgus ankle OA is posttraumatic. Osseous valgus deformities may result from severe ankle fracture with valgus impacted tibial plafond.[6,17,21] Moreover, patients with malunited fibula fracture with shortened and externally rotated fibula may present with asymmetric valgus ankle OA.[7,22,23] Chronic posttraumatic medial ankle instability is another etiologic factor in asymmetric valgus ankle OA.[5,24,25]

Table 1		
Etiologic groups of asymmetric arthritic valgus ankles			
Group	**Etiologic Factors**	
Primary	Posterior tibial tendon dysfunction Grade IV Talocalcaneal and/or calcaneonavicular coalition Pes planovalgus deformity	
Posttraumatic	Intra-articular ankle fracture with valgus impacted tibial plafond Fibular malunion with shortened and externally rotated fibula Chronic medial ankle instability	

BIOMECHANICS OF VALGUS ANKLE OSTEOARTHRITIS

While numerous studies have addressed the biomechanics of end-stage ankle OA,[26–28] there are limited data on asymmetric ankle OA. Asymmetric valgus ankle OA shows specific pathobiomechanical characteristics in the ankle joint (**Box 1, Fig. 1**).

Knupp and colleagues[9] used a cadaveric model to address the effect of valgus and varus supramalleolar level deformities on the pressure distribution in the tibiotalar joint. Specimens were divided into groups with and without fibular osteotomy. Of note, isolated valgus and varus supramalleolar deformity without fibula osteotomy led to a change in the force vector and shift of the peak pressure in the anteromedial and posterolateral direction, respectively. However, in specimens with fibula osteotomy the observed findings were different: there was a posterolateral shift for valgus deformity and an anteromedial shift for varus deformity. This study highlighted the complexity of asymmetric ankle OA with concomitant valgus or varus deformity.[9] Stufkens and colleagues[29] used 17 cadaveric lower legs in a biomechanical study to address the role of the fibula in varus and valgus deformity of the tibia. Surprisingly, a created supramalleolar valgus deformity did not lead to a lateral shift of intra-articular pressure distribution; rather, the opposite was observed because of the restricting role of the fibula.

Nuesch and colleagues[30] addressed kinematic and kinetic changes in 8 patients with asymmetric ankle OA in a comparison with 15 healthy individuals. A significant reduction in peak ground reaction force and peak kinetic values was observed in the OA group. Furthermore, patients with asymmetric ankle OA had a significantly lower dorsiflexion and rotation range of motion of the involved hindfoot.[30] In another study by the same group, muscle activation during isometric contractions and level walking was assessed in 12 patients with asymmetric ankle OA.[31] These patients showed pathologically altered patterns of muscle activation during gait, with a general shift toward lower activation frequencies and lower plantarflexion and dorsiflexion torques.

Davitt and colleagues[32] addressed the effect of inframalleolar alignment on ankle and subtalar joint pressure distribution by performing 1-cm medial and lateral displacement calcaneal osteotomies in 6 cadaver specimens. Only small effects on pressure distribution in the ankle and posterior facet of the subtalar joint were observed after translation osteotomies of the calcaneus.

Box 1
Pathobiomechanical characteristics of the asymmetric valgus ankle osteoarthritis

- Valgus hindfoot deformity

- Lateralized mechanical lower leg axis

- Asymmetric force vector of the triceps surae: lateralized pull of heel cord

- Tibiotalar joint: reduced contact area, increased lateral joint reaction/peak forces, lateral overload/overuse

- Overload of medial ankle ligaments: medial ligament complex deficiency

- Overstress of syndesmotic ligaments

- Lateral fibulocalcaneal impingement

- Lateral malleolus stress fracture

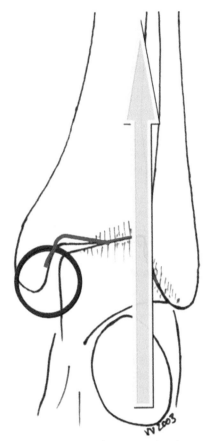

Fig. 1. Pathobiomechanical characteristics of asymmetric valgus ankle osteoarthritis. Lateralized mechanical lower leg axis (*yellow arrow*) inevitably leads to overload of lateral compartment of the tibiotalar joint (*red line*) and overload of medial ankle ligaments, with consecutive medial ligament complex deficiency (*blue circle*).

Despite the limited literature addressing biomechanics of asymmetric ankle OA, it has been clearly shown that supramalleolar deformities result in altered load distribution and, consequently, altered muscle activation to compensate for the asymmetric OA.

DIAGNOSIS OF VALGUS ANKLE OSTEOARTHRITIS
Clinical Assessment

Clinical assessment of patients with valgus ankle OA starts with careful review of patient history. All patients are asked if they have had prior trauma, conservative therapies or surgeries, concomitant disease, or infections. All medical reports and imaging studies should be collected and analyzed for patients with previous traumas and/or surgeries. The current status is evaluated, considering the following aspects. The level and type of actual pain (overall, waking, stressed, resting, night pain) is assessed, for which a visual analog scale (VAS) of 0 points (no pain) to 10 points (maximal pain) can be used.[33] The level of sports and recreation activity is assessed using the following scores: grade 0, none; grade 1, moderate, grade 2, normal; grade 3, high; and grade 4, elite.[34,35]

Ankle range of motion is measured clinically using a goniometer placed along the lateral border of the leg and foot with the patient in a weight-bearing position, as described by Lindsjö and colleagues.[36] Hindfoot stability is manually tested with the patient seated, using standard talar tilt stress tests (inversion stress test for lateral and eversion stress test for medial ankle instability) and anterior drawer tests.[37] Hindfoot alignment is judged from behind the patient who is in a weight-bearing position. The function of all tendons crossing the ankle joint is tested. The posterior tibial tendon function is assessed with a single heel-rise test by observing hindfoot inversion (variation of the heel).[38–40] In patients with posterior tibial tendon dysfunction, a Myerson classification system[41] or a novel, systematic RAM (rearfoot [R], ankle [A], or midfoot [M]) classification[40] should be used.

Radiographic Assessment

The authors routinely use 4 weight-bearing radiographs for radiographic assessment: lateral and dorsoplantar view of the foot, mortise view of the tibiotalar joint, and the Saltzman view. The Saltzman view[42] is indispensable in assessing inframalleolar alignment because visual judgment of hindfoot alignment is inaccurate.[43] In patients with concomitant deformities/abnormalities of the knee and/or hip, radiographs of the whole leg should also be performed. Single photon-emission computed tomography/computed tomography (SPECT-CT) is useful for localization of degenerative joint changes and their biological activity.[44,45] Furthermore, it has been shown that this diagnostic tool has a high sensitivity for assessment of osseous structures in patients with chronic foot and ankle pain.[46]

High-quality magnetic resonance imaging (MRI) (3 T, 1-mm slices) may also be useful for decision making, as it shows the amount of osteochondral degeneration and possible signs of coentities in valgus asymmetric ankle OA, such as medial ankle ligament lesions or posterior tibial tendon involvement.[47,48]

JOINT-PRESERVING SURGERY OF THE VALGUS OSTEOARTHRITIC ANKLE
Indications, Contraindications, Risks, and Pitfalls

The most common indication for joint-preserving surgery is asymmetric lateral ankle OA with a partially preserved medial compartment of the tibiotalar joint (**Table 2**).[7,8,14] The cartilage status of the medial compartment of the ankle joint should be confirmed using different imaging modalities including conventional weight-bearing radiographs, SPECT-CT, and MRI.[49] Another indication for realignment surgery is osteochondral lesions on the lateral aspect of the tibiotalar joint.[50,51] In such cases, the authors suggest cartilage reconstructive procedures (eg, repair of osteochondral lesions with the aid of modified autologous matrix-induced chondrogenesis) and realignment surgery of concomitant deformities.[50,51] In patients with posttraumatic deformities (malunions) of the lower leg, realignment surgery may restore the hindfoot biomechanics and postpone the further development of ankle OA.[8,22] In patients with end-stage ankle OA with concomitant valgus deformity, realignment surgery should be performed before or with ankle joint–sacrificing procedures such as total ankle replacement or ankle arthrodesis.[10,52,53] The general contraindications for realignment surgery include acute or chronic osteomyelitis or infection, and severe vascular and/or neurologic deficiency in the affected lower extremity. In heavy smokers a higher nonunion rate may be observed. The special contraindication for realignment joint-preserving surgery is end-stage ankle OA with degenerative involvement of more than half of the tibiotalar

Table 2
Indications, contraindications, special risks, and pitfalls for realignment surgery in patients with asymmetric valgus ankle osteoarthritis

Indications	Asymmetric lateral ankle osteoarthritis with concomitant valgus deformity with a medial partially preserved tibiotalar joint
	Osteochondral lesions on the talar aspect of the tibiotalar joint
	Corrections of posttraumatic deformities after lower leg fractures
	Hindfoot realignment before or together with ankle joint–sacrificing procedures (eg, total ankle replacement, ankle arthrodesis)
Contraindications	End-stage ankle osteoarthritis with involvement of more than half of the tibiotalar joint surface
	Unmanageable hindfoot instability
	Acute osteomyelitis or infection
	Severe vascular and/or neurologic deficiency
	Heavy smoking (because of most likely expected high rate of nonunion or delayed union)
	Relative contraindications:
	Advanced age (>70 y)
	Patients of poor general condition who are unable to perform postoperative non–weight-bearing rehabilitation
	Insulin-dependent diabetes (with or without diabetic polyneuropathy)
	Altered bone quality due to medication (eg, long-term medication with steroids)
	Large cysts
	Osteopenia or osteoporosis
	Rheumatoid osteoarthritis
Special risks	Intraoperative injury of neurovascular structures and/or tendons
	Wound-healing problems/infections
	Undercorrection/overcorrection
	Loss of correction
	Delayed union/nonunion
	Hardware removal because of pain/discomfort

joint surface and cases with progressive hindfoot instability, which cannot be addressed by ligamental reconstruction procedures. The relative contraindications are summarized in **Table 2**. The intraoperative and perioperative complications of realignment surgery include intraoperative injuries of neurovascular structures and/or tendons, and wound-healing problems or infections (see **Table 2**). A careful preoperative analysis of underlying deformity and surgical planning may help to avoid the undercorrection or overcorrection of deformity. Delayed union or nonunion may result from inappropriate fixation techniques or noncompliance in the early postoperative phase when only partial weight bearing is allowed. Loss of correction can be observed in patients with implant failure or in those in whom concomitant deformities and problems (eg, ligamental instability, inframalleolar deformities) have not been properly addressed. In patients with painful hardware, a hardware removal should be performed after osseous healing at the site of osteotomies has been achieved.

Treatment Algorithm

The aim of the treatment algorithm presented herein is to realign the hindfoot and shift the heel contact point from the concave side of the deformity to the convex side, resulting in a stable and parallel ankle space in the frontal plane.[8] Step-by-step procedures of the algorithm are shown in **Fig. 2**.

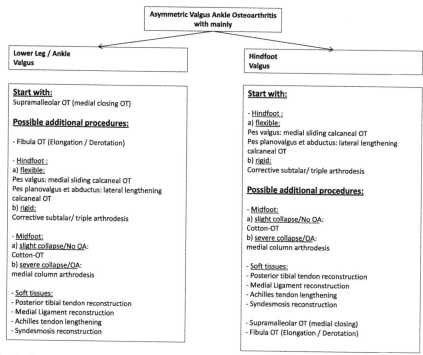

Fig. 2. Treatment algorithm of asymmetric valgus ankle osteoarthritis. OT, osteotomy.

Before realignment surgery, anterior ankle arthroscopy is recommended to assess the extent and degree of cartilage degeneration. If the valgus deformity is predominantly at or above the ankle joint (typical in posttraumatic cases), the first step is correction above the ankle joint (see **Fig. 2**). Tibia valgus malalignment is planned for slight overcorrection: the aim is a tibial surface angle of 85° to 90°. Significant overcorrection should be avoided, to limit shear forces across the realigned tibiotalar joint. In the second step, the necessity of osteotomy is assessed, first for the fibula and then for inframalleolar hindfoot deformity. For a flexible hindfoot deformity the authors perform hindfoot and midfoot osteotomies and add requisite medial soft-tissue procedures. In patients with a fixed hindfoot deformity with substantial degenerative changes of the subtalar and Chopart joint, a corrective subtalar or triple arthrodesis is suggested.

In a hindfoot valgus-driven lateral ankle degeneration, for example from a chronic posterior tibial tendon insufficiency, coalition, or chronic medial ankle instability, the joint-preserving surgery algorithm starts with correction of the hindfoot, (ie, inframalleolar), differentiating whether the hindfoot is flexible or rigid (see **Fig. 2**).

SUPRAMALLEOLAR MEDIAL CLOSING-WEDGE OSTEOTOMY

Supramalleolar realignment osteotomy is a relatively new surgical technique, introduced in 1995 by Takakura and colleagues.[54] Stamatis and colleagues[55] treated 22 patients (23 ankles) with supramalleolar osteotomies for painful distal tibial malalignment of at least 10° with or without radiographic evidence of ankle OA. All varus deformities were corrected using a medial opening-wedge osteotomy, and all valgus deformities with a medial closing-wedge osteotomy. In 2 patients secondary surgery was necessary because of the nonunion of the osteotomy. The remaining osteotomies healed within a mean time of 14 weeks. Significant improvement of American Ortho-paedic Foot and Ankle Society (AOFAS) score and Takakura ankle score was observed, with no differences regarding the surgical technique (opening-wedge vs closing-wedge).[55] Pagenstert and colleagues[8] reported midterm results obtained from 35 consecutive patients who underwent realignment surgery because of valgus or varus ankle OA. At the mean follow-up of 5 years, significant pain relief, functional improvement, and increased range of motion were observed. Revision was necessary in 10 ankles, including in 3 patients who underwent total ankle replacement.[8] Hinter-mann and colleagues[11] described the surgical technique of realignment surgery and presented outcomes in 74 patients. Forty-five patients had joint-preserving surgery because of substantial valgus malalignment of the hindfoot. The investigators pre-sented promising results whereby in most cases arthrodesis or total ankle replace-ment was postponed. Knupp and colleagues[13] reported on 92 patients (94 ankles) with asymmetric ankle OA, 61 of whom had valgus deformity. At the mean follow-up of 43 months a significant improvement in clinical scores was observed, with post-operative reduction of radiographic signs of OA in patients with midstage ankle OA. In 10 patients, conversion to total ankle replacement or arthrodesis was necessary owing to progression of ankle OA. Hintermann and colleagues[22] performed a prospective study including 48 patients with malunited, pronation-external rotation fracture of the ankle. In all patients, valgus malalignment of the distal tibia and malunion of the fibula were corrected. At a mean follow-up of 7.1 years, good or excellent results were obtained in 42 patients. In 1 patient total ankle replacement was performed 26 months after corrective surgery.

Preoperative Planning

The amount of surgical correction should be planned using weight-bearing anteropos-terior and lateral radiographs. One essential radiographic parameter in determining the supramalleolar varus or valgus deformity is the medial distal tibial angle.[56,57] In the previously published radiologic[57] and cadaver[56] studies this was measured as $92.4° \pm 3.1°$ (range, 84°–100°) and $93.3° \pm 3.2°$ (range, 88°–100°), respectively. Stufk-ens and colleagues[58] demonstrated that this angle differs between radiographs of the whole lower leg and mortise views of the ankle; therefore, it should be measured using standardized radiographs. Furthermore, substantial disagreement in primary supra-malleolar alignment (as measured using the medial distal tibial angle) was found be-tween the mortise and Saltzman views.[59] Talar tilt in the ankle mortise has been calculated as the difference between the medial distal tibial angle and the tibiotalar angle (normal value $91.5° \pm 1.2°$).[60] The limit for clinically relevant talar tilting was set at 4°.[13,61]

To determine the height of the wedge (H) to be removed, the width of the distal part of the tibia (W) is measured using a weight-bearing anteroposterior radiograph (**Fig. 3**). The following calculation determines the height of the wedge: $H = \tan \alpha_1 \times W$, with α_1 quantifying the amount of deformity with the desired overcorrection.[62,63] The proximal plane of the osteotomy is maintained perpendicular to the medial tibial cortex. The distal plane is planned on the basis of the height of the osteotomy wedge as described above.

Surgical Technique

The procedure can be performed under general or regional anesthesia. The patient is placed in a supine position. The ipsilateral leg is lifted until a strictly upward position of the foot is obtained. A tourniquet is applied on the ipsilateral thigh, with pressure not

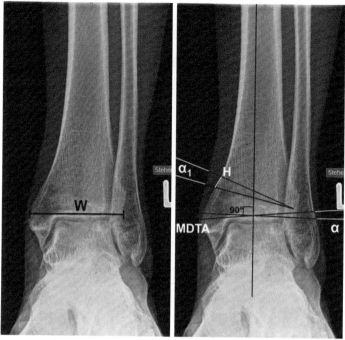

Fig. 3. Preoperative planning of a supramalleolar medial closing-wedge osteotomy. H, height of the wedge to be removed; MDTA, medial distal tibial angle; W, width of the distal part of the tibia; α, valgus deformity; α_1, amount of valgus deformity with desired overcorrection.

exceeding 350 mm Hg. In most patients anterior ankle arthroscopy is performed using standard portals.[64,65] Cartilage degeneration is assessed using the Outerbridge classification.[66] The authors use a medial approach with skin incision over the distal tibial and medial malleolus. After exposure of the distal tibia by incision of the periosteum, the plane of the osteotomy is determined using fluoroscopic image intensification. Two Kirschner wires are placed according to the preoperatively planned amount of correction. Before the osteotomy is performed, Hohmann retractors are used to protect the neurovascular and tendon structures of the anterior and posterior lower leg. The osteotomy is performed using an oscillating saw, with irrigation to reduce thermal damage that may impair the postoperative osseous healing. The osteotomy can be refined using a chisel to preserve the lateral cortex and improve the intrinsic stability of the osteotomy. The osteotomy is stabilized by an angular stable plate (eg, distal tibial locking compression plate [LCP], T-shaped 3.5-mm LCP) (**Fig. 4**). Eccentrically introduced cortical screws proximal to the osteotomy, or a tension device, can be used to increase the pressure at the site of the closed osteotomy.

FIBULA OSTEOTOMY

The incidence of distal fibula malunions after fibular reconstruction is up to 33%.[67] Distal fibula malunions with fibula shortening and external rotation with lateral talar tilt are problematic because they disrupt the congruency of the ankle mortise.[67] It has been shown that small displacements of the fibula (eg, 2 mm shortening, 2 mm lateral shift, or 5° of external rotation) may significantly increase the contact pressures of the tibiotalar joint.[68] Therefore, corrective distal fibular osteotomies may limit the

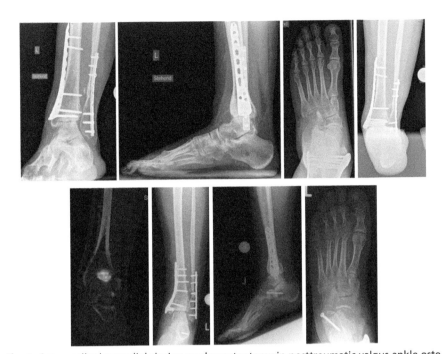

Fig. 4. Supramalleolar medial closing-wedge osteotomy in posttraumatic valgus ankle oste-oarthritis. Preoperative weight-bearing radiographs including Saltzman view show beginning degenerative changes of the lateral tibiotalar joint with valgus hindfoot alignment, abductus deformity of the midfoot and forefoot, and shortened and externally malrotated fibula in a patient 11 months after open reduction and internal fixation of bimalleolar fracture. Hardware removal, supramalleolar medial closing-wedge osteotomy, and lateral lengthening osteotomy of the calcaneus were performed to address the valgus tilt of the talus and pes planovalgus et abductus deformity.

progression of posttraumatic ankle OA.[67] Offierski and colleagues[69] performed a lengthening osteotomy in 11 patients, and stated that such reconstructive surgery may provide considerable functional and symptomatic improvement even long after the initial surgery. Similar results were observed by Ward and colleagues.[70] Weber and colleagues[71] performed lengthening osteotomy of the fibula in 7 patients with posttraumatic malunion whereby both a horizontal and Z-osteotomy of the fibula were used. Sinha and colleagues[72] performed a transverse fibular osteotomy, and used a tricortical iliac bone graft with fibular plate fixation in 7 patients with a malunited fibular fracture. Restoration of fibular length and the shape of the ankle mortise were achieved and no complications were observed.

Surgical Technique

First, fluoroscopy is used to assess the malrotation and length of the fibula. A longitudinal incision is made over the fibula. In patients with previous surgeries (eg, open reduction and internal fixation of fibula fractures), scar tissue at the anterior syndesmosis should be removed, but the syndesmotic ligaments should remain preserved to allow mobilization of the fibula. Z-shaped osteotomy of the fibula is performed using an oscillating saw. In patients with rotational deformity of the fibula, a bone wedge is removed for correction. After elongation and derotation of the fibula, the osteotomy is fixed with clamps and checked using fluoroscopy. Appropriate fibula position is defined by the following criteria[22]: (1) appropriate closure of the medial clear space with restoration of the medial gutter; (2) anatomic position of the talus within the mortise; and (3) restoration of anatomic landmarks as described by Weber and Simpson.[73] Final fixation of the fibula osteotomy is performed using 1 or 2 lag screws and a 3.5-mm LCP angular stable plate.

MEDIAL SLIDING CALCANEAL OSTEOTOMY

For correction of hindfoot and midfoot valgus, 3 types of osteotomy are available: medial sliding calcaneal osteotomy, lateral lengthening calcaneal osteotomy, and Cotton osteotomy (**Table 3**). Depending on the 3-dimensional correction effect, 1 of the 3 osteotomies is selected. Sometimes a combination of 2 or of all 3 is necessary to correct the hindfoot or midfoot.

Calcaneal osteotomy was first described in 1893 by Gleich as a treatment option for correction of pes planovalgus deformity.[74,75] In the 1960s Dwyer described his surgical technique comprising a lateral opening-wedge osteotomy using a tibial bone graft. The main indication for medial sliding calcaneal osteotomy is the correction of the hindfoot valgus deformity and redirection of the coronal vector of the Achilles tendon.[76] Some cadaver studies address the biomechanics of medial displacement calcaneal osteotomy. Steffensmeier and colleagues[77] measured tibiotalar joint contact stresses to investigate the effects of medial and lateral displacement calcaneal osteotomies. In 8 cadaver specimens a 1-cm medial displacement shifted the center of pressure an average of 1.58 mm medially at the applied load of 1330 N.[77] Hadfield and colleagues[78] showed that medial displacement calcaneal osteotomy with 1-cm medial translation did not lead to a significant increase in the length of Achilles tendon. In another study the same group addressed the effects of medial sliding calcaneal osteotomy, with and without superior translation, on Achilles tendon elongation and plantar foot pressures.[79] The addition of a 0.5-cm superior translation to the osteotomy allowed off-loading of the medial forefoot without increasing lateral forefoot or heel pressures.[79] Arangio and Salathe[80] demonstrated that a 10-mm medial sliding calcaneal osteotomy may substantially decrease the load on the first metatarsal and the moment at the talonavicular joint while increasing the load on the fifth metatarsal and the calcaneal-cuboid joint.

Koutsogiannis[81] was one of the first to reintroduce the medial sliding calcaneal osteotomy for correction of pes planovalgus deformity. Several clinical studies have demonstrated encouraging results after this procedure.[15,74,82–91]

Surgical Technique

The lateral calcaneal wall is exposed using a small, oblique skin incision approximately 2 cm posterior and parallel to the peroneal tendons. Special attention should

Table 3			
Calcaneal and midfoot osteotomies and their correction effect			
Correction Effect	Medial Sliding Calcaneal OT	Lateral Lengthening Calcaneal OT	Cotton OT
Heel variation	+++	++	−
Forefoot adduction	+	+++	+
Medial arch restoration	+	++	+++

Abbreviation: OT, osteotomy.

be paid to avoid injury to the sural nerve and its branches. Dorsal and plantar borders of the calcaneus are identified and protected using 2 Hohmann retractors. The osteotomy is performed using an oscillating saw, and an osteotome can be used to complete the osteotomy on the medial aspect. A large laminar spreader is used for stepwise mobilization of osteotomy fragments. After appropriate mobilization and relaxation of the surrounding soft tissues, the calcaneal tuber can be medialized as preoperatively planned using the Saltzman view.[42] Cranial dislocation of the distal fragment should be avoided. If the desired medialization cannot be achieved, the dislocation maneuver should be repeated with a plantarflexed ankle and flexed knee to relax the entire calf musculature. The position of the tuber calcanei is preliminarily stabilized using 2 Kirschner wires. After confirmation by fluoroscopy, final fixation is performed using 1 or 2 6.5-mm cannulated headless compression screws (**Fig. 5**).

LATERAL LENGTHENING CALCANEAL OSTEOTOMY

Lateral lengthening calcaneal osteotomy is used with a medializing calcaneal osteotomy and a distraction calcaneocuboid arthrodesis to treat adult flatfoot deformity.[92]

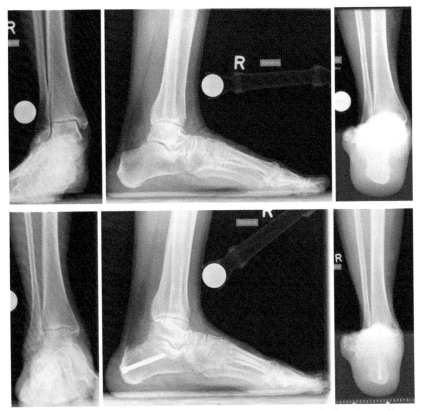

Fig. 5. Medial sliding osteotomy of the calcaneus. Preoperative weight-bearing radiographs including Saltzman view (*top*) show severe valgus malalignment of the hindfoot and substantial flattening of the medial arch. Postoperative weight-bearing radiographs (*bottom*) show completely healed calcaneus osteotomy and physiologic alignment of the hindfoot at the follow-up of 2 years.

Evans[93] originally described this procedure with osteotomy localization approximately 1.5 cm parallel to and distal to the calcaneocuboid joint. Raines and Brage[94] performed an anatomic study to identify the safest osteotomy level. The lateral lengthening calcaneal osteotomy was performed 5, 10, and 15 mm from the joint. The investigators concluded that a 10-mm interval is the safest option by which to avoid injury to both the anterior and middle facets of the subtalar joint. Hintermann and colleagues[95,96] modified the Evans osteotomy by 12 to 18 mm proximal to the calcaneocuboid joint and by crossing the calcaneus along the posterior facet, avoiding violations of the subtalar articular surfaces. Thomas and colleagues[97] compared the lateral lengthening calcaneal osteotomy with calcaneocuboid distraction arthrodesis in 27 and 17 feet, respectively. The functional outcome was comparable, but major complications were observed more often in the arthrodesis group, including 2 nonunions and 3 delayed unions. Haeseker and colleagues[98] performed a similar comparative study including 14 patients with distraction arthrodesis and 19 who underwent lateral lengthening calcaneal osteotomy. Postoperatively, the patients in the osteotomy group had better functional results as assessed using AOFAS score and comparable radiographic outcome. The rate of postoperative complications was comparable in both groups. The ideal graft size was identified to be between 8 and 12 mm, in most cases 10 mm.[97,99–101] Both graft types (allograft or autograft) can be used to fill the osteotomy gap.[92] Dolan and colleagues[102] performed a randomized study including 33 feet in 31 patients to compare iliac crest autograft with allograft in lateral lengthening calcaneal osteotomy. In all feet, complete osseous union was observed. Of note, after 8 weeks 94% of grafts united in the allograft group, whereas only 60% of autografts had united by the same time. Grier and Walling[103] compared both types of graft in calcaneocuboid arthrodesis and lateral lengthening calcaneal osteotomy, with 94% union observed in the allograft group and 70% in autograft group. In both groups platelet-rich plasma was used additionally.[103]

Surgical Technique

The authors use a lateral approach for lateral lengthening calcaneus osteotomy. A horizontal incision is made below the level of the sinus tarsi. The fat pad of the sinus tarsi is held dorsally with a Hohmann hook, and the posterior facet of the subtalar joint is exposed. Another Hohmann retractor is placed between calcaneal lateral wall and peroneal tendons. The lateral calcaneal wall osteotomy is performed using an oscillating saw at the level of the floor of the sinus tarsi. The medial calcaneal cortex should be preserved. A spreader is placed over the osteotomy and the osteotomy is mobilized until the pes planovalgus et abductus deformity of the hindfoot, midfoot, and forefoot is sufficiently corrected. The lateral osteotomy gap (typically between 8 and 14 mm) can be filled using allograft or autograft (eg, iliac crest autograft). The osteotomy can be fixed using a 3.5-mm cortical AO screw inserted from distal into the posteromedial calcaneus (**Fig. 6**). As an alternative, in patients with reduced bone quality a small plate can be used for osteotomy fixation.

FIRST CUNEIFORM OPENING DORSAL WEDGE (COTTON) OSTEOTOMY

In patients with moderate break of the medial arch or forefoot supinatus without midfoot OA, a first cuneiform opening dorsal wedge osteotomy, or Cotton osteotomy, should be performed. This procedure was first described in 1936.[104] In patients with stage II posterior tibial tendon dysfunction, the main indication for Cotton osteotomy is a persistent forefoot varus deformity without instability or arthritis of the first tarsometatarsal (TMT) or metatarsal-cuneiform joints.[105] Bruyn and colleagues[106] treated

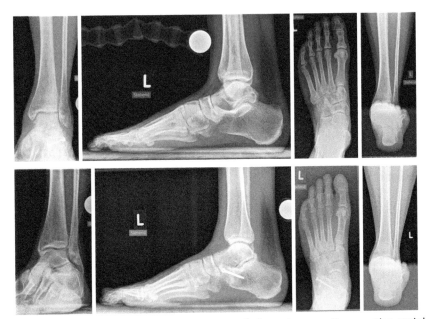

Fig. 6. Lateral column lengthening osteotomy of the calcaneus. Preoperative weight-bearing radiographs including Saltzman view (*top*) show substantial abductus deformity of the midfoot and valgus malalignment of the hindfoot. Postoperative weight-bearing radiographs (*bottom*) show complete osseous integration of allograft at the site of the calcaneal osteotomy and physiologic alignment of the midfoot and hindfoot at the follow-up of 1 year.

20 patients (25 feet) with symptomatic severe flexible pes planovalgus deformity by a combination of Evans calcaneal osteotomy and subtalar joint arthroereisis. In 9 feet the Cotton osteotomy was also performed. A subjective questionnaire revealed that all patients were very satisfied with the postoperative results, with an average score of 93 based on a 100-point scale. Hirose and Johnson[107] addressed the effectiveness of the Cotton osteotomy in 16 feet (15 patients) with flatfoot deformities of several causes including congenital flatfoot, tarsal coalition, overcorrected clubfoot deformity, skewfoot, chronic posterior tibial tendon insufficiency, and rheumatoid arthritis. The investigators detected a substantial improvement in radiographic parameters, and no nonunions or malunions were observed. In a cadaver study, Scott and colleagues[108] used lower extremities to measure plantar pressures after Cotton osteotomy, and showed that the Cotton osteotomy leads to increased pressures within the medial forefoot, although a significant compensatory decrease in lateral forefoot pressure was not observed. League and colleagues[109] performed a biomechanical cadaver study for radiographic and pedobarographic comparison of femoral head allograft versus block plate in Cotton osteotomy. In specimens with a block plate procedure, the calcaneal pitch was significantly lower. The pedobarographic investigations showed increased medial and decreased lateral pressures. Yarmel and colleagues[110] performed a thorough literature review, and described the surgical technique of the Cotton osteotomy as a powerful surgical tool in the treatment of severe pes planovalgus deformity with persistent rigid forefoot varus deformity. Lutz and Myerson[111] reported on outcomes of the Cotton osteotomy in 101 cases. No nonunions were observed. A significant improvement in the Meary angle, from a

preoperative average value of −23° to an average postoperative value of −1°, was observed. Recently, McCormick and Johnson[112] reviewed medial column procedures in the correction of adult acquired flatfoot deformity, and stated that this powerful procedure may correct residual forefoot varus, allowing preservation the joints of the first foot ray.

Surgical Technique

A small incision is performed dorsomedially over the first cuneiform bone. The osteotomy site is marked with a Kirschner wire and is performed using a small oscillating saw blade or chisel. After opening the osteotomy, the gap is filled with allograft or autograft (eg, iliac crest graft). Final fixation is performed using a small angular stable dorsal plate.

MEDIAL COLUMN ARTHRODESIS

In cases of midfoot collapse, forefoot supinatus, or osteoarthritic medial column joints, plantarflexing medial column arthrodesis might be necessary to restore the medial foot arch; for example, naviculocuneiform arthrodesis, first TMT arthrodesis (modified or original Lapidus arthrodesis), or a complete midfoot medial column arthrodesis.

SOFT-TISSUE RECONSTRUCTIONS
Posterior Tibial Tendon Reconstruction

Flexor digitorum longus transfer
The posterior tibial tendon (PTT) is exposed using a medial approach. The PTT is inspected visually and by palpation for any pathologic changes including tears, tenosynovitis, or thickening. Degenerative changes of the tendon should be carefully debrided. The flexor digitorum longus (FDL) is identified posterolateral to the PTT. The sheath of FDL is dissected and the FDL is mobilized in maximal eversion of the foot. The authors prefer FDL transfer with side-to-side suturing to the PTT without creating a transnavicular tunnel.

Cobb procedure
The PTT is exposed using a medial approach, and all degenerative changes of the tendon are carefully debrided. For the harvesting of the anterior tibial tendon, a 2- to 3-cm incision 5 cm above the extensor retinaculum is made. The anterior tibial tendon is split using a scalpel, and the middle third of the tendon is dissected as far proximal as possible. The graft is rerouted using a long curved clamp. The free end of the graft is attached to the proximal end of the PTT using side-to-side sutures over the entire length of the tendon while the foot is in a forced supination and plantarflexion position.

Medial Ankle Ligament Reconstruction
Surgical exploration of the medial ankle ligament is performed through a 4- to 8-cm skin incision, starting 1 to 2 cm above the medial malleolus tip toward the medial aspect of the navicular bone. The anterior aspect of the deltoid ligament is exposed by dissection of the fascia. The sheath of the PTT is longitudinally incised, and tendon is carefully checked. After the exploration of the PTT, the spring ligament is identified and inspected, then the tibionavicular and tibiospring ligaments are explored. In most cases, anatomic repair and reattachment should be performed. The anterior border of the medial malleolus is exposed by a short longitudinal incision between the

tibionavicular and tibiospring ligaments. The surface of the medial aspect is roughened with a rongeur. Reattachment of the ligament can be performed using an anchor or transosseous sutures. If necessary, nonresorbable sutures are placed in the spring ligament. The tibionavicular and spring ligaments are further stabilized using resorbable sutures. In cases with significant degenerative changes of the ligament, a plantaris graft technique can be used.[113]

SUMMARY

Patients with substantial valgus or varus deformity often present with pathologically altered pressure distribution patterns in the tibiotalar joint,[9,114–116] resulting in development of asymmetric ankle OA. Realignment surgery may restore normal biomechanics of the ankle joint, resulting in substantial postoperative pain relief, functional improvement, and slowing of the degeneration process.[8,22,54,117] Depending on the origin and classification of the valgus deformity, the authors recommend a step-by-step treatment algorithm, including osseous corrective procedures on the supramalleolar and inframalleolar level and soft-tissue reconstruction procedures. One of the main advantages of realignment surgery is that it is a joint-preserving procedure. Most patients show high satisfaction with the surgery,[8,22] even allowing them to return to normal sports and recreation activities.[35] In cases with degenerative changes of the tibiotalar joint requiring a second surgery (total ankle replacement or ankle arthrodesis), patients may also benefit from the realignment surgery. It has been shown that total ankle replacement performed in a well-aligned hindfoot has a better postoperative outcome.[53,118–121] Overall, promising short-term and mid-term results have been observed in patients who underwent realignment surgery because of substantial valgus deformity. Further long-term clinical studies should be performed to address positive and negative predictors that influence the long-term success after this surgery.

REFERENCES

1. Glazebrook M, Daniels T, Younger A, et al. Comparison of health-related quality of life between patients with end-stage ankle and hip arthrosis. J Bone Joint Surg Am 2008;90(3):499–505.
2. Anderson DD, Chubinskaya S, Guilak F, et al. Post-traumatic osteoarthritis: improved understanding and opportunities for early intervention. J Orthop Res 2011;29(6):802–9.
3. Saltzman CL, Salamon ML, Blanchard GM, et al. Epidemiology of ankle arthritis: report of a consecutive series of 639 patients from a tertiary orthopaedic center. Iowa Orthop J 2005;25:44–6.
4. Valderrabano V, Horisberger M, Russell I, et al. Etiology of ankle osteoarthritis. Clin Orthop Relat Res 2009;467(7):1800–6.
5. Valderrabano V, Hintermann B, Horisberger M, et al. Ligamentous posttraumatic ankle osteoarthritis. Am J Sports Med 2006;34(4):612–20.
6. Horisberger M, Valderrabano V, Hintermann B. Posttraumatic ankle osteoarthritis after ankle-related fractures. J Orthop Trauma 2009;23(1):60–7.
7. Pagenstert G, Knupp M, Valderrabano V, et al. Realignment surgery for valgus ankle osteoarthritis. Oper Orthop Traumatol 2009;21(1):77–87.
8. Pagenstert GI, Hintermann B, Barg A, et al. Realignment surgery as alternative treatment of varus and valgus ankle osteoarthritis. Clin Orthop Relat Res 2007; 462:156–68.

9. Knupp M, Stufkens SA, van Bergen CJ, et al. Effect of supramalleolar varus and valgus deformities on the tibiotalar joint: a cadaveric study. Foot Ankle Int 2011; 32(6):609–15.

10. Valderrabano V, Frigg A, Leumann A, et al. Total ankle arthroplasty in valgus ankle osteoarthritis. Orthopade 2011;40(11):971–7 [in German].

11. Hintermann B, Knupp M, Barg A. Osteotomies of the distal tibia and hindfoot for ankle realignment. Orthopade 2008;37(3):212–3 [in German].

12. Horn DM, Fragomen AT, Rozbruch SR. Supramalleolar osteotomy using circular external fixation with six-axis deformity correction of the distal tibia. Foot Ankle Int 2011;32(10):986–93.

13. Knupp M, Stufkens SA, Bolliger L, et al. Classification and treatment of supramalleolar deformities. Foot Ankle Int 2011;32:1023–31.

14. Barg A, Pagenstert GI, Leumann AG, et al. Treatment of the arthritic valgus ankle. Foot Ankle Clin 2012;17(4):647–63.

15. Myerson MS, Badekas A, Schon LC. Treatment of stage II posterior tibial tendon deficiency with flexor digitorum longus tendon transfer and calcaneal osteotomy. Foot Ankle Int 2004;25(7):445–50.

16. Francisco R, Chiodo CP, Wilson MG. Management of the rigid adult acquired flatfoot deformity. Foot Ankle Clin 2007;12(2):317–27.

17. Bluman EM, Chiodo CP. Valgus ankle deformity and arthritis. Foot Ankle Clin 2008;13(3):443–70.

18. Bluman EM, Myerson MS. Stage IV posterior tibial tendon rupture. Foot Ankle Clin 2007;12(2):341–62, viii.

19. Bohay DR, Anderson JG. Stage IV posterior tibial tendon insufficiency: the tilted ankle. Foot Ankle Clin 2003;8(3):619–36.

20. Thorpe SW, Wukich DK. Tarsal coalitions in the adult population: does treatment differ from the adolescent? Foot Ankle Clin 2012;17(2):195–204.

21. McCann PA, Jackson M, Mitchell ST, et al. Complications of definitive open reduction and internal fixation of pilon fractures of the distal tibia. Int Orthop 2011;35(3):413–8.

22. Hintermann B, Barg A, Knupp M. Corrective supramalleolar osteotomy for malunited pronation-external rotation fractures of the ankle. J Bone Joint Surg Br 2011;93(10):1367–72.

23. van Wensen RJ, van den Bekerom MP, Marti RK, et al. Reconstructive osteotomy of fibular malunion: review of the literature. Strategies Trauma Limb Reconstr 2011;6(2):51–7.

24. Hintermann B. Medial ankle instability. Foot Ankle Clin 2003;8(4):723–38.

25. Hintermann B, Valderrabano V, Boss A, et al. Medial ankle instability: an exploratory, prospective study of fifty-two cases. Am J Sports Med 2004; 32(1):183–90.

26. Barton T, Lintz F, Winson I. Biomechanical changes associated with the osteoarthritic, arthrodesed, and prosthetic ankle joint. Foot Ankle Surg 2011;17(2):52–7.

27. von Tscharner V, Valderrabano V. Classification of multi muscle activation patterns of osteoarthritis patients during level walking. J Electromyogr Kinesiol 2010;20(4):676–83.

28. Valderrabano V, Nigg BM, von Tscharner V, et al. Gait analysis in ankle osteoarthritis and total ankle replacement. Clin Biomech (Bristol, Avon) 2007;22(8): 894–904.

29. Stufkens SA, van Bergen CJ, Blankevoort L, et al. The role of the fibula in varus and valgus deformity of the tibia: a biomechanical study. J Bone Joint Surg Br 2011;93(9):1232–9.

30. Nuesch C, Valderrabano V, Huber C, et al. Gait patterns of asymmetric ankle osteoarthritis patients. Clin Biomech (Bristol, Avon) 2012;27(6):613–8.

31. Nuesch C, Huber C, Pagenstert G, et al. Muscle activation of patients suffering from asymmetric ankle osteoarthritis during isometric contractions and level walking—a time-frequency analysis. J Electromyogr Kinesiol 2012;22:939–46.

32. Davitt JS, Beals TC, Bachus KN. The effects of medial and lateral displacement calcaneal osteotomies on ankle and subtalar joint pressure distribution. Foot Ankle Int 2001;22(11):885–9.

33. Huskisson EC. Measurement of pain. Lancet 1974;2(7889):1127–31.

34. Valderrabano V, Pagenstert G, Horisberger M, et al. Sports and recreation activity of ankle arthritis patients before and after total ankle replacement. Am J Sports Med 2006;34(6):993–9.

35. Pagenstert G, Leumann A, Hintermann B, et al. Sports and recreation activity of varus and valgus ankle osteoarthritis before and after realignment surgery. Foot Ankle Int 2008;29(10):985–93.

36. Lindsjö U, Danckwardt-Lilliestrom G, Sahlstedt B. Measurement of the motion range in the loaded ankle. Clin Orthop Relat Res 1985;199(199):68–71.

37. Phisitkul P, Chaichankul C, Sripongsai R, et al. Accuracy of anterolateral drawer test in lateral ankle instability: a cadaveric study. Foot Ankle Int 2009;30(7):690–5.

38. Van Boerum DH, Sangeorzan BJ. Biomechanics and pathophysiology of flat foot. Foot Ankle Clin 2003;8(3):419–30.

39. Brilhault J, Noel V. PTT functional recovery in early stage II PTTD after tendon balancing and calcaneal lengthening osteotomy. Foot Ankle Int 2012;33(10):813–8.

40. Raikin SM, Winters BS, Daniel JN. The RAM classification: a novel, systematic approach to the adult-acquired flatfoot. Foot Ankle Clin 2012;17(2):169–81.

41. Myerson MS. Adult acquired flatfoot deformity: treatment of dysfunction of the posterior tibial tendon. Instr Course Lect 1997;46:393–405.

42. Saltzman CL, el Khoury GY. The hindfoot alignment view. Foot Ankle Int 1995;16(9):572–6.

43. Frigg A, Nigg B, Davis E, et al. Does alignment in the hindfoot radiograph influence dynamic foot-floor pressures in ankle and tibiotalocalcaneal fusion? Clin Orthop Relat Res 2010;468(12):3362–70.

44. Knupp M, Pagenstert GI, Barg A, et al. SPECT-CT compared with conventional imaging modalities for the assessment of the varus and valgus malaligned hindfoot. J Orthop Res 2009;27(11):1461–6.

45. Pagenstert GI, Barg A, Leumann AG, et al. SPECT-CT imaging in degenerative joint disease of the foot and ankle. J Bone Joint Surg Br 2009;91(9):1191–6.

46. Kretzschmar M, Wiewiorski M, Rasch H, et al. ^{99m}Tc-DPD-SPECT/CT predicts the outcome of imaging-guided diagnostic anaesthetic injections: a prospective cohort study. Eur J Radiol 2011;80(3):e410–5.

47. Chhabra A, Soldatos T, Chalian M, et al. Current concepts review: 3T magnetic resonance imaging of the ankle and foot. Foot Ankle Int 2012;33(2):164–71.

48. Gyftopoulos S, Bencardino JT. Normal variants and pitfalls in MR imaging of the ankle and foot. Magn Reson Imaging Clin N Am 2010;18(4):691–705.

49. Leumann A, Valderrabano V, Plaass C, et al. A novel imaging method for osteochondral lesions of the talus–comparison of SPECT-CT with MRI. Am J Sports Med 2011;39(5):1095–101.

50. Valderrabano V, Miska M, Leumann A, et al. Reconstruction of osteochondral lesions of the talus with autologous spongiosa grafts and autologous matrix-induced chondrogenesis. Am J Sports Med 2013;41(3):519–27.

51. Wiewiorski M, Barg A, Valderrabano V. Autologous matrix-induced chondrogenesis in osteochondral lesions of the talus. Foot Ankle Clin 2013;18:151–8.
52. Kim BS, Knupp M, Zwicky L, et al. Total ankle replacement in association with hindfoot fusion: outcome and complications. J Bone Joint Surg Br 2010; 92(11):1540–7.
53. Knupp M, Stufkens SA, Bolliger L, et al. Total ankle replacement and supramalleolar osteotomies for malaligned osteoarthritis ankle. Tech Foot & Ankle 2010;9: 175–81.
54. Takakura Y, Tanaka Y, Kumai T, et al. Low tibial osteotomy for osteoarthritis of the ankle. Results of a new operation in 18 patients. J Bone Joint Surg Br 1995; 77(1):50–4.
55. Stamatis ED, Cooper PS, Myerson MS. Supramalleolar osteotomy for the treatment of distal tibial angular deformities and arthritis of the ankle joint. Foot Ankle Int 2003;24(10):754–64.
56. Inman VT. The joints of the ankle. Baltimore (MD): Williams & Wilkins; 1976.
57. Knupp M, Ledermann H, Magerkurth O, et al. The surgical tibiotalar angle: a radiologic study. Foot Ankle Int 2005;26(9):713–6.
58. Stufkens SA, Barg A, Bolliger L, et al. Measurement of the medial distal tibial angle. Foot Ankle Int 2011;32:288–93.
59. Barg A, Harris MD, Henninger HB, et al. Medial distal tibial angle: comparison between weightbearing mortise view and hindfoot alignment view. Foot Ankle Int 2012;33(8):655–61.
60. Tanaka Y, Takakura Y, Fujii T, et al. Hindfoot alignment of hallux valgus evaluated by a weightbearing subtalar x-ray view. Foot Ankle Int 1999;20(10):640–5.
61. Cox JS, Hewes TF. "Normal" talar tilt angle. Clin Orthop Relat Res 1979;140: 37–41.
62. Knupp M, Barg A, Bolliger L, et al. Reconstructive surgery for overcorrected clubfoot in adults. J Bone Joint Surg Am 2012;94(15):e1101–7.
63. Warnock KM, Johnson BD, Wright JB, et al. Calculation of the opening wedge for a low tibial osteotomy. Foot Ankle Int 2004;25(11):778–82.
64. Golano P, Vega J, Perez-Carro L, et al. Ankle anatomy for the arthroscopist. Part I: the portals. Foot Ankle Clin 2006;11(2):253–73.
65. Golano P, Vega J, Perez-Carro L, et al. Ankle anatomy for the arthroscopist. Part II: role of the ankle ligaments in soft tissue impingement. Foot Ankle Clin 2006;11(2):275–96.
66. Outerbridge RE. The etiology of chondromalacia patellae. J Bone Joint Surg Br 1961;43:752–7.
67. Chu A, Weiner L. Distal fibula malunions. J Am Acad Orthop Surg 2009;17(4): 220–30.
68. Thordarson DB, Motamed S, Hedman T, et al. The effect of fibular malreduction on contact pressures in an ankle fracture malunion model. J Bone Joint Surg Am 1997;79(12):1809–15.
69. Offierski CM, Graham JD, Hall JH, et al. Late revision of fibular malunion in ankle fractures. Clin Orthop Relat Res 1982;171:145–9.
70. Ward AJ, Ackroyd CE, Baker AS. Late lengthening of the fibula for malaligned ankle fractures. J Bone Joint Surg Br 1990;72(4):714–7.
71. Weber D, Friederich NF, Muller W. Lengthening osteotomy of the fibula for post-traumatic malunion. Indications, technique and results. Int Orthop 1998;22(3): 149–52.
72. Sinha A, Sirikonda S, Giotakis N, et al. Fibular lengthening for malunited ankle fractures. Foot Ankle Int 2008;29(11):1136–40.

73. Weber BG, Simpson LA. Corrective lengthening osteotomy of the fibula. Clin Orthop Relat Res 1985;199(199):61–7.
74. Guha AR, Perera AM. Calcaneal osteotomy in the treatment of adult acquired flatfoot deformity. Foot Ankle Clin 2012;17(2):247–58.
75. Haddad SL, Myerson MS, Younger A, et al. Symposium: adult acquired flatfoot deformity. Foot Ankle Int 2011;32(1):95–111.
76. Giza E, Cush G, Schon LC. The flexible flatfoot in the adult. Foot Ankle Clin 2007; 12(2):251–71.
77. Steffensmeier SJ, Saltzman CL, Berbaum KS, et al. Effects of medial and lateral displacement calcaneal osteotomies on tibiotalar joint contact stresses. J Orthop Res 1996;14(6):980–5.
78. Hadfield MH, Snyder JW, Liacouras PC, et al. Effects of medializing calcaneal osteotomy on Achilles tendon lengthening and plantar foot pressures. Foot Ankle Int 2003;24(7):523–9.
79. Hadfield M, Snyder J, Liacouras P, et al. The effects of a medializing calcaneal osteotomy with and without superior translation on Achilles tendon elongation and plantar foot pressures. Foot Ankle Int 2005;26(5):365–70.
80. Arangio GA, Salathe EP. A biomechanical analysis of posterior tibial tendon dysfunction, medial displacement calcaneal osteotomy and flexor digitorum longus transfer in adult acquired flat foot. Clin Biomech (Bristol, Avon) 2009;24(4): 385–90.
81. Koutsogiannis E. Treatment of mobile flat foot by displacement osteotomy of the calcaneus. J Bone Joint Surg Br 1971;53(1):96–100.
82. Stufkens SA, Knupp M, Hintermann B. Medial displacement calcaneal osteotomy. Tech Foot & Ankle 2009;8:85–90.
83. Pomeroy GC, Manoli A. A new operative approach for flatfoot secondary to posterior tibial tendon insufficiency: a preliminary report. Foot Ankle Int 1997;18(4): 206–12.
84. Pinney SJ, Lin SS. Current concept review: acquired adult flatfoot deformity. Foot Ankle Int 2006;27(1):66–75.
85. Fayazi AH, Nguyen HV, Juliano PJ. Intermediate term follow-up of calcaneal osteotomy and flexor digitorum longus transfer for treatment of posterior tibial tendon dysfunction. Foot Ankle Int 2002;23(12):1107–11.
86. Wacker JT, Hennessy MS, Saxby TS. Calcaneal osteotomy and transfer of the tendon of flexor digitorum longus for stage-II dysfunction of tibialis posterior. Three- to five-year results. J Bone Joint Surg Br 2002;84(1):54–8.
87. Guyton GP, Jeng C, Krieger LE, et al. Flexor digitorum longus transfer and medial displacement calcaneal osteotomy for posterior tibial tendon dysfunction: a middle-term clinical follow-up. Foot Ankle Int 2001;22(8):627–32.
88. Hockenbury RT, Sammarco GJ. Medial sliding calcaneal osteotomy with flexor hallucis longus transfer for the treatment of posterior tibial tendon insufficiency. Foot Ankle Clin 2001;6(3):569–81.
89. Sammarco GJ, Hockenbury RT. Treatment of stage II posterior tibial tendon dysfunction with flexor hallucis longus transfer and medial displacement calcaneal osteotomy. Foot Ankle Int 2001;22(4):305–12.
90. Niki H, Hirano T, Okada H, et al. Outcome of medial displacement calcaneal osteotomy for correction of adult-acquired flatfoot. Foot Ankle Int 2012;33(11): 940–6.
91. Kou JX, Balasubramaniam M, Kippe M, et al. Functional results of posterior tibial tendon reconstruction, calcaneal osteotomy, and gastrocnemius recession. Foot Ankle Int 2012;33(7):602–11.

92. Roche AJ, Calder JD. Lateral column lengthening osteotomies. Foot Ankle Clin 2012;17(2):259–70.
93. Evans D. Calcaneo-valgus deformity. J Bone Joint Surg Br 1975;57(3):270–8.
94. Raines RA Jr, Brage ME. Evans osteotomy in the adult foot: an anatomic study of structures at risk. Foot Ankle Int 1998;19(11):743–7.
95. Hintermann B, Valderrabano V. Lateral column lengthening by calcaneal osteotomy. Tech Foot & Ankle 2003;2:84–90.
96. Hintermann B, Valderrabano V, Kundert HP. Lengthening of the lateral column and reconstruction of the medial soft tissue for treatment of acquired flatfoot deformity associated with insufficiency of the posterior tibial tendon. Foot Ankle Int 1999;20(10):622–9.
97. Thomas RL, Wells BC, Garrison RL, et al. Preliminary results comparing two methods of lateral column lengthening. Foot Ankle Int 2001;22(2):107–19.
98. Haeseker GA, Mureau MA, Faber FW. Lateral column lengthening for acquired adult flatfoot deformity caused by posterior tibial tendon dysfunction stage II: a retrospective comparison of calcaneus osteotomy with calcaneocuboid distraction arthrodesis. J Foot Ankle Surg 2010;49(4):380–4.
99. Pomeroy GC, Pike RH, Beals TC, et al. Acquired flatfoot in adults due to dysfunction of the posterior tibial tendon. J Bone Joint Surg Am 1999;81(8): 1173–82.
100. Tien TR, Parks BG, Guyton GP. Plantar pressures in the forefoot after lateral column lengthening: a cadaver study comparing the Evans osteotomy and calcaneocuboid fusion. Foot Ankle Int 2005;26(7):520–5.
101. Iaquinto JM, Wayne JS. Effects of surgical correction for the treatment of adult acquired flatfoot deformity: a computational investigation. J Orthop Res 2011; 29(7):1047–54.
102. Dolan CM, Henning JA, Anderson JG, et al. Randomized prospective study comparing tri-cortical iliac crest autograft to allograft in the lateral column lengthening component for operative correction of adult acquired flatfoot deformity. Foot Ankle Int 2007;28(1):8–12.
103. Grier KM, Walling AK. The use of tricortical autograft versus allograft in lateral column lengthening for adult acquired flatfoot deformity: an analysis of union rates and complications. Foot Ankle Int 2010;31(9):760–9.
104. Cotton FJ. Foot statics and surgery. N Engl J Med 1936;214:353–62.
105. Tankson CJ. The Cotton osteotomy: indications and techniques. Foot Ankle Clin 2007;12(2):309–15, vii.
106. Bruyn JM, Cerniglia MW, Chaney DM. Combination of Evans calcaneal osteotomy and STA-Peg arthroereisis for correction of the severe pes valgo planus deformity. J Foot Ankle Surg 1999;38(5):339–46.
107. Hirose CB, Johnson JE. Plantarflexion opening wedge medial cuneiform osteotomy for correction of fixed forefoot varus associated with flatfoot deformity. Foot Ankle Int 2004;25(8):568–74.
108. Scott AT, Hendry TM, Iaquinto JM, et al. Plantar pressure analysis in cadaver feet after bony procedures commonly used in the treatment of stage II posterior tibial tendon insufficiency. Foot Ankle Int 2007;28(11):1143–53.
109. League AC, Parks BG, Schon LC. Radiographic and pedobarographic comparison of femoral head allograft versus block plate with dorsal opening wedge medial cuneiform osteotomy: a biomechanical study. Foot Ankle Int 2008; 29(9):922–6.
110. Yarmel D, Mote G, Treaster A. The Cotton osteotomy: a technical guide. J Foot Ankle Surg 2009;48(4):506–12.

111. Lutz M, Myerson M. Radiographic analysis of an opening wedge osteotomy of the medial cuneiform. Foot Ankle Int 2011;32(3):278–87.
112. McCormick JJ, Johnson JE. Medial column procedures in the correction of adult acquired flatfoot deformity. Foot Ankle Clin 2012;17(2):283–98.
113. Pagenstert GI, Hintermann B, Knupp M. Operative management of chronic ankle instability: plantaris graft. Foot Ankle Clin 2006;11(3):567–83.
114. Ting AJ, Tarr RR, Sarmiento A, et al. The role of subtalar motion and ankle contact pressure changes from angular deformities of the tibia. Foot Ankle 1987;7(5):290–9.
115. Tarr RR, Resnick CT, Wagner KS, et al. Changes in tibiotalar joint contact areas following experimentally induced tibial angular deformities. Clin Orthop Relat Res 1985;199:72–80.
116. Wagner KS, Tarr RR, Resnick C, et al. The effect of simulated tibial deformities on the ankle joint during the gait cycle. Foot Ankle 1984;5(3):131–41.
117. Takakura Y, Takaoka T, Tanaka Y, et al. Results of opening-wedge osteotomy for the treatment of a post-traumatic varus deformity of the ankle. J Bone Joint Surg Am 1998;80(2):213–8.
118. Brunner S, Knupp M, Hintermann B. Total ankle replacement for the valgus unstable osteoarthritic ankle. Tech Foot & Ankle 2010;9:165–74.
119. Kim BS, Choi WJ, Kim YS, et al. Total ankle replacement in moderate to severe varus deformity of the ankle. J Bone Joint Surg Br 2009;91(9):1183–90.
120. Kim BS, Lee JW. Total ankle replacement for the varus unstable osteoarthritic ankle. Tech Foot & Ankle 2010;9:157–67.
121. Wood PL, Deakin S. Total ankle replacement. The results in 200 ankles. J Bone Joint Surg Br 2003;85(3):334–41.

Joint-Preserving Surgery of Asymmetric Ankle Osteoarthritis with Peritalar Instability

Beat Hintermann, MD[a],*, Markus Knupp, MD[a], Alexej Barg, MD[b]

KEYWORDS

- Peritalar instability • Varus ankle • Valgus ankle • Asymmetric ankle osteoarthritis
- Joint-preserving surgery • Supramalleolar osteotomy • Calcaneal osteotomy

KEY POINTS

- Meticulous clinical and radiographic assessment of the foot and ankle is mandatory for recognition of peritalar instability.
- Peritalar instability is a main cause of coronal plane instability of talus.
- Supramalleolar and inframalleolar correcting osteotomies are mainstays for successful treatment.
- Additional soft tissue procedure are, in most instances, required to get a stable and balanced ankle.

INTRODUCTION

The most common cause of end-stage osteoarthritis of the ankle is previous trauma.[1,2] Newer studies have shown that in up to 60% of affected ankles, with progression of osteoarthritic process, the talus did experience a varus or valgus tilt within the ankle mortise.[2–5] The underlying mechanism of this phenomenon is not well understood. One reason may be a concomitant peritalar instability, which allows the talus to translate and rotate on the calcaneus.[6]

This article discusses the anatomic and biomechanical properties of the asymmetrically osteoarthritic ankle with peritalar instability; it also presents an overview of indications and the technique of surgical procedures for joint-preserving reconstruction in these complex conditions.

Disclosures: B.H. has received royalty payments from Integra.
[a] Orthopaedic Department, Clinic of Orthopaedic Surgery and Traumatology, Kantonsspital Baselland, Rheinstrasse 26, Liestal CH-4410, Switzerland; [b] Orthopaedic Department, University Hospital of Basel, Spitalstrasse 21, Basel CH-4031, Switzerland
* Corresponding author.
E-mail address: beat.hintermann@ksbh.ch

ANATOMY AND BIOMECHANICS

The ankle consists of 3 bones: the tibia, the fibula, and the talus. The distal tibia and fibula form the mortise or proximal concave surface of the ankle joint. The body of the talus with its convex surface is held within the mortise. The distal tibial plafond has a concave shape, with an average medial angle of $22° \pm 4°$, and shows a slight varus.[7] The mean distal tibial angle (the angle between the longitudinal axis of the tibia and the plafond of the tibia) is approximately 93°, with a range between 84° and 100°.[8] The talus articulates with the tibia superiorly and medially, and with the fibula laterally. The talus has a conically shaped surface, with a smaller medial radius and medially directed apex. The joint surfaces have been shown to provide as much as 100% stability of the talus within the ankle mortise while the foot is loaded.[9] This characteristic, in turn, may suggest that incompetence of collateral ligaments does not affect talar position within the ankle.

The subtalar joint has complex anatomy and consists of 3 articulating facets: anterior, intermediate-anterior, and posterior.[10] Whereas the posterior facet of the subtalar joint has a convex/concave surface like a ball-and-socket joint, the anterior facet of the subtalar joint shows a more flat configuration.[6,11] With this configuration, the subtalar joint allows rotational movements, which particularly support accommodation during walking or running on uneven ground, and also translational movements, which allow the talus in addition to move medially and laterally, and anteriorly and posteriorly.

Besides joint surfaces, complex ligament structures provide stability to the talus, including the collateral ligaments of the ankle joint complex, and the interosseous ligament. The talus itself has no tendon insertions, and therefore, its position cannot be influenced directly by activation of periarticular muscles. However, the joint-crossing extrinsic tendons and muscles may play an important role in active stabilization of the hindfoot. With its sandwichlike position, the talus is controlled and manipulated by forces applied from proximal and distal segments. Under physiologic conditions, there is an equilibrium of acting forces supported by intrinsic stability of the tibiotalar joint. In cases without the contribution of the intrinsic stability of the tibiotalar joint, the subtalar joint seems not to be able to compensate for instability and may start to tilt, resulting in peritalar instability.

The talus may tilt, with progressive joint load, into varus or valgus, depending on the load pattern resulting from deformity or incompetence of ligament structures (**Fig. 1**). In most cases, the calcaneus goes in the opposite direction, resulting in a so-called zigzag or Z-shaped deformity. This contradictory movement of the calcaneus may often result in a clinical appearance of a well-aligned hindfoot. Because its height has decreased, the surrounding soft tissue structures do typically show additional loss of tension, with the clinical appearance of a floppy foot. In parallel, containment forces of articular surfaces decrease. The complexity of undergoing deformation processes is a major challenge for reconstruction surgery, and success depends on to what extent the surgeon is able to identify and address the underlying problems.

INDICATIONS FOR JOINT-PRESERVING SURGERY

Joint-preserving treatments aim to reduce symptoms and to diminish harmful influences on the joint mechanics, which may slow down or even stop the degenerative process. Indications for joint-preserving surgery include bony and soft tissue balancing procedures, such as correcting supramalleolar and inframalleolar osteotomies, ligament reconstructions, tendon transfers, and selected arthrodesis in a nonarthritic or early-stage osteoarthritic ankle with preserved range of motion. The contraindications are end-stage osteoarthritis, severe unmanageable hindfoot

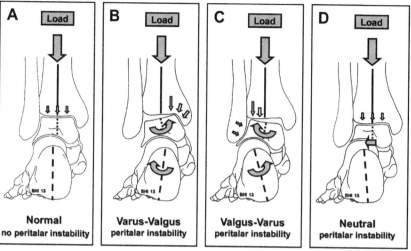

Fig. 1. Influence of loading and force pattern to the tibiotalar joint in the ankle joint complex without and with peritalar instability: (*A*) balanced joint; (*B*) varus-valgus ankle; (*C*) valgus-varus ankle; and (*D*) neutral ankle with translational peritalar instability.

instability, severe vascular or neurologic deficiency in the affected extremity, and neuropathic disorders (eg, Charcot arthropathy). Relative contraindications that need to be considered are altered bone quality (because of medication, large cysts, and osteopenia or osteoporosis), older age (>70 years), insulin-dependent diabetes, smoking, and rheumatic disease.

PREOPERATIVE PLANNING

The most important aspect of preoperative planning is assessment of the origin of the deformity, and the understanding of deformation forces. It is mandatory to separate the different types of deformities, in particular of varus and valgus tilted talar deformities, which can be a deviation mainly in the coronal plane but also in the sagittal plane.

Clinical Examination

Physical examination includes clinical assessment of the hindfoot while the patient is standing. In some patients, the valgus or varus deformity can be observed only under physiologic load. Typically, the deformity does increase under loading. Toe walking may help to evaluate the calcaneus position. Hindfoot stability needs to be assessed with routine physical examination. The function of joint-crossing tendons is tested, in particular the peroneal tendons in the varus ankle, and the posterior tibial tendon in the valgus ankle. The range of motion of the ankle joint is measured clinically using a goniometer placed along the lateral border of the leg and foot.[12] The forefoot is assessed with regard to a plantarflexed first ray, forefoot supination, and toe deformities.

Radiographic Examination

Radiographic assessment of peritalar instability includes anteroposterior (AP), lateral, and mortise views of the ankle and the dorsoplantar view of the foot. All radiographs should be performed with weight-bearing to assess the functional deformities of the hindfoot. In order to assess the calcaneus position in relationship to the longitudinal axis of the tibia, the Saltzman view (hindfoot alignment view) should be performed.[13] Single-photon emission computed tomography may be helpful for the understanding of deformity and planning of osteotomies, particularly in biplanar corrections.[14]

Based on the tilting pattern of the talus within the mortise, peritalar instability can be classified mainly into varus and valgus types, but the talus can also remain in a neutral position.[6] In all deformity types, the talus can, in the sagittal plane, remain in its proper position or move into dorsiflexion or plantarflexion, combined with or without translation in the AP direction. In each of these types, the talus can, in the horizontal plane, remain in its proper position relative to the calcaneus, or rotate internally or externally, respectively.

Planning of Correction

Before surgery, the correction is planned on the AP and lateral view radiographs. The tibial articular surface (TAS) angle (normal value, 91°–93°) is measured. The lateral view radiographs are used to distinguish between patients who present with a centered joint and those with an anterior extrusion of the talus out of the mortise. The Saltzman view is used to assess overall alignment of the hindfoot.

Supramalleolar osteotomies

The aims of supramalleolar osteotomies are to realign the hindfoot, to transfer the ankle joint under the weight-bearing axis, and to normalize the direction of the force vector of the triceps surae.[15,16] An open or closing wedge osteotomy from medially or laterally, or, in severe deformities, a domelike osteotomy from anteriorly can be considered to achieve an overcorrection of 2° to 5°. A fibular osteotomy, solely or in addition to tibial correcting osteotomy, can be considered to address malpositioning that may hinder reduction of talus (eg, shortening, lengthening, derotation, or abduction).[17]

Inframalleolar osteotomies

The aims of inframalleolar osteotomies are to realign the hindfoot, and to normalize the direction of the force vector of the triceps surae. A medial or lateral sliding osteotomy or a lateral closing wedge osteotomy can be considered to achieve a neutral alignment of the hindfoot.

Osteotomies of the medial arch

The aims of osteotomies at the medial arch are to realign the forefoot to the hindfoot. In the case of forefoot supination, a dorsal closing wedge osteotomy of the first cuneiform or the base of the first metatarsal is considered, whereas in the case of forefoot pronation, a dorsal opening wedge osteotomy of the first cuneiform is considered.

Talocalcaneal (subtalar) arthrodesis

The aims of a subtalar arthrodesis are to correct a fixed deformity, to stabilize a highly unstable joint, or to address pain originating from progressive degenerative changes. In most instances, an interposition technique with the use of bone graft should be considered in order to tighten the collapsed ligaments of the ankle joint complex.

Tarsal arthodesis

The aims of tarsal arthrodesis are to realign the forefoot to the hindfoot, to stabilize the medial arch, and to address pain originating from degenerative changes. Depending on the origin of the problem, the arthrodesis can be considered at the level of talonavicular, naviculocuneiform, or first tarsometatarsal joints. The goal is to obtain a neutral position of the forefoot.

Ligament reconstructions

The aims of ligament reconstructions are to stabilize the talus in a corrected position within the ankle mortise. Anatomic repair of remaining ligament can be augmented with the use of free tendon autografts, (eg, plantaris tendon or semitendinosus tendon). If available, the use of allografts can also be considered. Although effective for stabilization of the ankle joint complex, tenodesis techniques should not be used, because they change the biomechanics and limit motion.

Tendon transfers

The aims of tendon transfers are to restore and to balance muscular forces. In the case of a dysfunction of the peroneal brevis, a peroneus longus to peroneus brevis tendon transfer is considered. In the case of a dysfunction of the tibialis posterior, a flexor digitorum longus to tibialis posterior tendon transfer is considered.

SURGICAL TECHNIQUE

Fluoroscopic assessment can be performed in the outpatient clinic and should then be repeated under anesthesia before surgery. With passive manipulation and valgus or valgus stress, the extent of correction of the talar position and the amount of lateral and medial instability can be assessed. The effect of segmental correction can be tested by insertion of percutaneous K-wires into the distal tibia and talus, respectively (**Fig. 2**). Distraction on the medial or lateral side can be used to evaluate the effect of tensioning of the ligaments on reorientation of the talus, or to identify a contracture of the subtalar joint. If the talus cannot be fully corrected within the ankle mortise, the underlying cause should be carefully identified.

Varus Ankle

In the varus type of peritalar instability, the talus is in a varus tilted position within the mortise, which typically increases while loading the foot as a result of rotational movement on the calcaneus. Its position in the sagittal and horizontal plane may also have changed. Although the lateral ligaments are almost always incompetent, the peroneal brevis tendon may also be incompetent. Neutral heel alignment may be preserved, but, in most instances, there is some varus misalignment though opposite valgus movement at the subtalar joint, which results in a zigzag deformity. The main problems are the anterolateral extrusion of the talus, and the wearing out of the medial tibial

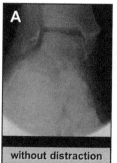
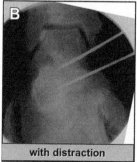
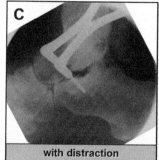

Fig. 2. Joint distraction through percutaneously inserted K-wires. (*A*) Valgus tilt of talus within the mortise, without distraction. With distraction, the proper position of the talus is obtained in the coronal plane (*B*) and sagittal plane (*C*).

plafond and medial malleolus with a round medial malleolus, both of which may render proper repositioning and stabilization of the talus within the mortise difficult.

In the case of a varus TAS angle, a medial opening wedge osteotomy of the tibia is aimed at obtaining 2° to 4° of valgus at TAS angle.[15,16] Through a medial approach, the distal tibia is exposed without stripping of the periosteum. A K-wire is used to determine the plane of the osteotomy under fluoroscopy. Subsequently, the osteotomy is performed using a wide saw blade, and the correction is made according to the preoperative plan. In the case of anterior extrusion, the correction is carried out in a biplanar fashion to improve the talar coverage in the anterior-posterior direction.[16] A bone autograft or allograft is used to fill the gap, and rigid plate fixation with interlocking screws is used to obtain a stable fixation. If the TAS is impacted significantly, resulting in more than 5° of varus of the medial joint, an intra-articular osteotomy might be considered instead.[18]

After the distal tibia osteotomy has been performed, the ankle mortise is checked under fluoroscopy. Talar reduction can be hindered by a medial soft tissue contracture (eg, deltoid ligament or posterior tibial contracture), bone formation in the lateral compartment of the ankle, or a too-long or malpositioned fibula (**Fig. 3**). In the case of medial soft tissue contracture, a release is performed until appropriate correction of talus is obtained. In the case of bone formation, cheilectomy is performed. In the case of inadequate length or position of fibula, the fibula is osteotomized and the position and length of the fibula adjusted.

As evaluated preoperatively, with a subtalar contracture or an extensive subtalar instability that may not be sufficiently addressed by ligament reconstruction, a subtalar arthrodesis is performed through a lateral approach to the sinus tarsi. After debridement of the articular surfaces to subchondral bone, fluoroscopy is used to obtain meticulous repositioning of the talus with regard to the calcaneus in all planes. K-wires are used for preliminary fixation, and 2 to 3 screws for final rigid fixation.

The lateral ligaments are exposed through a lateral incision. If detached from the fibula, as is the case in most instances, the ligaments are prepared for reattachment by

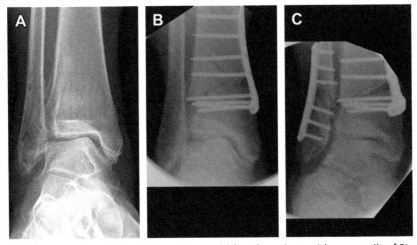

Fig. 3. (*A*) Varus-valgus deformity in a 54 year-old female patient, with a varus tilt of 8° preoperatively. (*B*) The talar tilt did not change after medial opening wedge osteotomy of the distal tibia because the mortise was too narrow. (*C*) Correcting fibular osteotomy did allow proper repositioning of the talus.

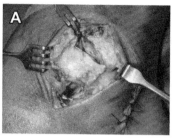
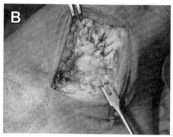

Fig. 4. (*A*) The lateral ankle ligaments are typically disattached from the fibula. (*B*) Strong reconstruction after reattachment to the fibula by a bony anchor or transosseous sutures.

the use of bony anchor or transosseous sutures (**Fig. 4**). A free tendon graft can also be used for anatomic reconstruction.[19] The peroneal tendons are then explored. In the case of an incompetent peroneal brevis tendon, as typically seen in elongation or ruptures, the peroneus longus tendon is exposed through a separate incision at the level of the cuboid bone. After dissection, it is fixed to the base of the fifth metatarsal while holding the foot in slight eversion and dorsiflexion, and the tendon is in addition (or additionally) fixed by side-to-side sutures to the peroneal brevis tendon (**Fig. 5**).[20] Thereafter, the ligament reconstruction is completed with sutures.

The alignment of the heel is reassessed clinically. The aim is to achieve a heel with 1° to 5° valgus. Any remaining deformity is addressed with an osteotomy of the calcaneus. The tuber calcanei are exposed through an oblique incision. A straight[21] or Z-shaped[22] osteotomy is performed with the use of a saw and chisels, and the tuber is then moved medially or laterally as necessary. One or 2 screws are used for rigid fixation.

The position of the forefoot is checked by holding the foot in neutral position. In the case of a plantarflexed first ray, the first cuneiform or base of first metatarsal is exposed through a dorsal approach. A closing wedge osteotomy is performed to achieve appropriate correction of the forefoot.[23]

Valgus Ankle

In the valgus type of peritalar instability, the talus has moved in a valgus tilted position within the mortise, which typically increases while loading the foot as a result of

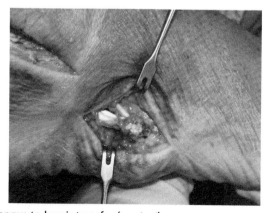

Fig. 5. Peroneal longus to brevis transfer (*see text*).

rotational movement on the calcaneus (**Fig. 6**). Its position in the sagittal and horizontal plane may also have changed. The medial ligaments can be, but must not be, incompetent, as is the case when the talus has impacted into the lateral tibial plafond. Neutral heel alignment may be preserved, but, in most instances, there is some valgus misalignment through opposite valgus movement at the subtalar joint, which results in a zigzag deformity. The main problems are the anterolateral impaction of the talus into anterolateral tibial plafond, and the incompetence of deep layers of deltoid ligaments (eg, talocalcaneal ligaments).

In the case of a valgus TAS angle, a medial closing wedge osteotomy of the tibia is aimed at obtaining 2° to 4° of varus at the TAS angle.[15–17] Through a medial approach, the distal tibia is exposed without stripping of the periosteum. Two K-wires are used to determine the 2 planes of the osteotomy under fluoroscopy, according to the preoperative plan. Subsequently, the osteotomy is performed using a wide saw blade and the osteotomy is closed by manual force. A rigid plate fixation with interlocking screws is used to obtain a stable fixation.

After completion of distal tibia osteotomy, the ankle mortise is checked under fluoroscopy. Talar reduction can be hindered by bone formation at the anterolateral edge of the tibia, or by sticking to a malpositioned fibula.[17] In the case of bone formation, cheilectomy is performed. In the case of inadequate length or position of the fibula, the fibula is osteotomized and the position and length of the fibula adjusted until the talus has moved into the correct position.[17,24]

As evaluated preoperatively, with a subtalar contracture or an extensive subtalar instability that may not be sufficiently addressed by ligament reconstruction, a subtalar arthrodesis is performed through a lateral approach to the sinus tarsi. Joint distraction over 2 K-wires is used. After debridement of the articular surfaces to subchondral bone, fluoroscopy is used to obtain meticulous repositioning of the talus with regard to the calcaneus in all planes. Joint distraction is typically applied to keep the ligaments tight (see **Fig. 2**). After the gap is filled with solid bone graft, K-wires are used for preliminary fixation, and 2 to 3 full-treated screws for rigid fixation (**Fig. 7**).

The medial ligaments (**Fig. 8**A) and the posterior tibial tendon (see **Fig. 8**B) are exposed through a medial incision. If disattached from the medial malleolus, as is the case in most instances, they are prepared for reattachment by the use of bony anchor or transosseous sutures.[25] If a posterior tibial dysfunction was evident in preoperative clinical assessment, the tendon is explored. If confirmed, a transfer of the flexor digitorum tendon is considered by fixation to the medial tuberosity of navicular bone by the use of an anchor, and additional side-to-side sutures to the distal aspect of the posterior tibial tendon are applied (see **Fig. 8**C).[26,27] In the case of poor quality of soft

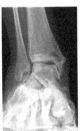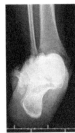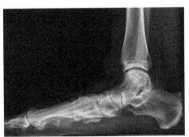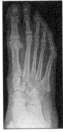

Fig. 6. Standard radiographs in the right foot of a 51-year-old female patient showing severe peritalar instability with valgus destabilization of the ankle joint complex and breakdown of the medial arch.

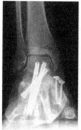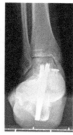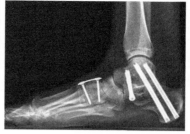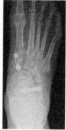

Fig. 7. Well-aligned and stable ankle joint complex after distraction arthrodesis of the subtalar joint and medial sliding osteotomy of the calcaneus (same patient as **Fig. 6**, 4 years after surgery).

tissue , a free tendon graft can also be used for reconstruction of the deltoid ligament (**Fig. 9**).

The lateral ankle stability is tested clinically and under fluoroscopy. If there is a lateral opening of the ankle joint, which is often the case, the lateral ankle ligament is exposed through a separate lateral approach. If disattached from the fibula, as is the case in most instances, they are reattached by the use of bony anchor or transosseous sutures. A free tendon graft can also be used for anatomic reconstruction.[28] The peroneal tendons are also explored. In the case of instability with subluxation or complete dislocation of peroneal tendons, the tendon sheath is reconstructed. In the case of a rupture, the tendon is reconstructed.

The alignment of the heel is reassessed clinically. The aim is to achieve a heel in a neutral or slightly varus position. Any remaining deformity is addressed with an osteotomy of the calcaneus (**Fig. 10**). The tuber calcanei are exposed through an oblique incision. The osteotomy is performed with the use of a saw and chisels, and the tuber is then moved medially as necessary. One or 2 screws are used for rigid fixation.[21]

The position of the forefoot is checked by holding the foot in a neutral position. In the case of distinct forefoot supination, which does not allow the foot to obtain full support of the first metatarsal head, a plantarflexion osteotomy is performed at the level of the first cuneiform. After having achieved the desired correction, a bone graft is used to fill the gap, and screw or plate fixation is used to ensure stability. In the case of a substantial forefoot supination or marked sag at the navicular-cuneiform or tarsometatarsal level, a correcting osteotomy[23] (**Fig. 11**) or arthrodesis[29] is performed. Usually, arthrodesis at the talonavicular is avoided to preserve some transverse joint motion to the foot.

Neutral ankle

In the neutral type of peritalar instability, the talus has not changed its position in the coronal plane, but in the sagittal and horizontal plane as a result of translational

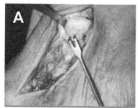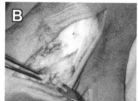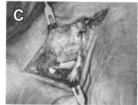

Fig. 8. Step-by step exploration of medial soft tissues shows a complete avulsion of superficial deltoid ligament (*A*) and a complete rupture of posterior tibial tendon (*B*). (*C*) Reconstruction of deltoid ligament and flexor digitorum tendon transfer (same patient as **Fig. 6**).

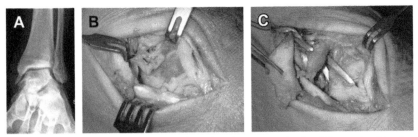

Fig. 9. (A) Valgus-varus deformity in a high-level gymnast (male, 26 years) with chronic rupture of deltoid ligament. (B) Surgical exposure showing a severe insufficiency of the deltoid ligament complex, including its superficial and deep layers. (C) A doubled free plantaris tendon graft was used for anatomic reconstruction.

movement on the calcaneus. Neutral heel alignment is normally preserved. The main problems are loss of height of the ankle joint complex, which, in turn, causes a relative attenuation of the ligaments because of the collapse and anterior ankle pain because of dorsiflexed position of talus.

The subtalar joint is approached through an incision to the sinus tarsi. Joint distraction with a K-wire in the neck of the talus and another one in the lateral calcaneus is

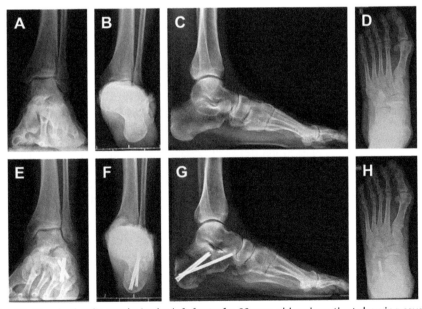

Fig. 10. Standard radiographs in the left foot of a 66 year-old male patient showing severe peritalar instability with valgus destabilization of the ankle joint complex associated with valgus malalignment of the heel and abduction of forefoot. (A) AP view of the ankle showing valgus tilt of talus; (B) Saltzman view showing a marked heel valgus; (C) lateral view of the ankle showing the peritalar instability; and (D) AP view of the foot showing an abduction of the forefoot. Eight weeks after double osteotomy of the calcaneus (medial sliding and lateral column lengthening), the ankle is balanced, and heel and foot alignment are restored (E–H). Notice that the medial and lateral ligaments of the ankle were also reconstructed.

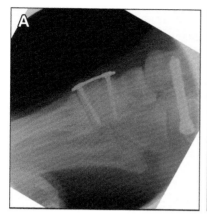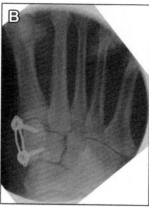

Fig. 11. An opening wedge osteotomy of the first cuneiform is used to plantarflex the first ray, thereby provide medial forefoot support beneath the first metatarsal. (*A*) Lateral view and (*B*) AP view (same patient as **Fig. 6**).

used to restore the talocalcaneal angle in the sagittal and horizontal plane. The subtalar joint is typically widely opened. After debridement to the subchondral bone, bone graft is used to fill the gap. Two parallel K-wires in the posterior aspect and another one in the anterior aspect of the subtalar joint are inserted under fluoroscopy, and 3 full-treated screws are used for final rigid fixation in a 3-pod manner.

Usually, no additional procedures have to be considered apart from interposition arthrodesis. In the case of remaining lateral ankle instability, ligament reconstruction is performed as described for the varus and valgus types.

Postoperative management
Patients are placed in a below-knee splint for 2 weeks followed by a removable walker with instructions to remain partially weight-bearing but to perform range-of-motion exercises. In the case of additional soft tissue reconstruction, a lower leg plaster may be used. Once bone healing is achieved, usually after 8 weeks, full weight-bearing is permitted, and a specific rehabilitation program is started.

COMPLICATIONS

Intraoperative complications include nerve injuries. An important consideration, especially with acute corrections, is the posterior tibial nerve. Varus-to-valgus corrections stretch this nerve, particularly if the center of rotation of angulation is distal to the osteotomy line. Acute tarsal tunnel syndrome can result from acute varus-to-valgus correction. A prophylactic tarsal tunnel release may be indicated for such acute corrections, especially in cases with previous scarring.

Overcorrection or undercorrection may occur after inappropriate preoperative planning, or, if fluoroscopy is not used for meticulous control of aimed cuts. An overcorrection of 2° to 3° is recommended by most investigators for asymmetric arthritis. Inappropriate removal of osteophytes may cause impingement and may also avoid appropriate repositioning of talus in the mortise.

Delayed or nonunion may result from inappropriate fixation techniques, or too aggressive loading of the leg in the early postoperative phase. Loss of correction may occur as a result of implant failure, or inappropriate addressing of concomitant problems such as ligamentous incompetence, muscular dysfunction, and forefoot deformities.

RESULTS AFTER JOINT-PRESERVING SURGERY

Although several reports have shown good to excellent survival rates and improvement in clinical outcomes after supramalleolar osteotomy in the asymmetric varus arthritic ankle,[15,16,30–32] only a few reports are available about the results for the asymmetric valgus arthritic ankle.[15,17,31] However, none of these reports has focused on loss of peritalar stability, which allows the talus to rotate and translate on calcaneal and navicular bone surfaces, thereby resulting in a three-dimensional positional change and various talar malpositioning, as the origin of the problem to be treated. No report exists about reconstructive surgery of talar malposition after loss of peritalar stability without supramalleolar correction.

Takakura and colleagues[32] described relief of pain and reduction of limitations in daily activities in 9 patients who underwent realignment surgery because of varus deformity of the ankle. Cheng and colleagues[30] reported on a selected series of 18 patients with low tibial osteotomies. These investigators obtained good or excellent results in all patients at a mean follow-up of 48 months. Pagenstert and colleagues[31] reported on a series of 35 patients who underwent supramalleolar osteotomies and found that total ankle replacement or ankle fusion was postponed in 91% of cases by realignment surgery. Most recently, Knupp and colleagues[15] confirmed these findings in 94 ankles and found significant improvement in the AOFAS (American Orthopaedic Foot and Ankle Society) hindfoot score and significant reduction in pain in the various types of asymmetric ankle osteoarthritis ($P<.05$).

Hintermann and colleagues[17] reported on a selected series of 48 patients with correction of a valgus deformity with corrective supramalleolar osteotomy of the ankle after malunited pronation-external rotation fractures of the ankle. These investigators emphasized the importance of correcting osteotomy of the fibula to achieve proper reduction of talus within the mortise. At a mean follow-up of 7.1 years, good or excellent results were obtained in 42 patients (87.5%), with the benefit being maintained over time. However, in these patients, the underlying cause was a malunited fracture and not a peritalar instability.

Reduction in signs of arthritis on plain radiographs after supramalleolar osteotomy has been described in several studies.[15–17,30–34] Knupp and colleagues[15] found a significant reduction ($P<.05$) in radiologic signs of arthritis in ankles presenting with talar tilt, whereas only tendencies were evident for the congruent joints. These changes were independent of age and gender.[15]

SUMMARY

Careful radiographic assessment of talar position in all 3 planes is mandatory for success in treatment of asymmetric varus or valgus arthritic ankles. Because articular surfaces may be worn out, isolated ligament reconstruction on the medial and lateral side of the ankle joint may not restore proper position of the talus within the ankle mortise. Osseous balancing with osteotomies above or below the ankle, or subtalar fusion, may thus be the main step for successful restoration of talar position within the ankle mortise. Meticulous reorientation of the forefoot and, if necessary, stabilization of the medial arch are also mandatory for long-term success of surgical reconstruction. Overall, the key for success is to use all treatment modalities necessary to restore appropriate alignment of the hindfoot complex. However, to further improve success in surgical reconstruction of the asymmetric arthritic ankle, more work is needed to better understand the ongoing processes in peritalar instability.

REFERENCES

1. Saltzman CL, Salamon ML, Blanchard GM, et al. Epidemiology of ankle arthritis: report of a consecutive series of 639 patients from a tertiary orthopaedic center. Iowa Orthop J 2005;25:44–6.
2. Valderrabano V, Horisberger M, Russell I, et al. Etiology of ankle osteoarthritis. Clin Orthop Relat Res 2009;467:1800–6.
3. Hayashi K, Tanaka Y, Kumai T, et al. Correlation of compensatory alignment of the subtalar joint to the progression of primary osteoarthritis of the ankle. Foot Ankle Int 2008;29:400–6.
4. Horisberger M, Valderrabano V, Hintermann B. Posttraumatic ankle osteoarthritis after ankle-related fractures. J Orthop Trauma 2009;23:60–7.
5. Lee WC, Moon JS, Lee HS, et al. Alignment of ankle and hindfoot in early stage ankle osteoarthritis. Foot Ankle Int 2011;32:693–9.
6. Hintermann B, Knupp M, Barg A. Peritalar instability. Foot Ankle Int 2012;33:450–4.
7. Inman VT, editor. The joints of the ankle. Baltimore (MD): Williams & Wilkins; 1976.
8. Knupp M, Ledermann H, Magerkurth O, et al. The surgical tibiotalar angle: a radiologic study. Foot Ankle Int 2005;26:713–6.
9. Stormont DM, Morrey BF, An KN, et al. Stability of the loaded ankle. Relation between articular restraint and primary and secondary static restraints. Am J Sports Med 1985;13:295–300.
10. Sarrafian SK. Biomechanics of the subtalar joint complex. Clin Orthop Relat Res 1993;(290):17–26.
11. Barg A, Tochigi Y, Amendola A, et al. Subtalar instability: diagnosis and treatment. Foot Ankle Int 2012;33:151–60.
12. Lindsjo U, Danckwardt-Lilliestrom G, Sahlstedt B. Measurement of the motion range in the loaded ankle. Clin Orthop Relat Res 1985;(199):68–71.
13. Saltzman CL, el Khoury GY. The hindfoot alignment view. Foot Ankle Int 1995;16: 572–6.
14. Knupp M, Pagenstert GI, Barg A, et al. SPECT-CT compared with conventional imaging modalities for the assessment of the varus and valgus malaligned hindfoot. J Orthop Res 2009;27:1461–6.
15. Knupp M, Stufkens SA, Bolliger L, et al. Classification and treatment of supramalleolar deformities. Foot Ankle Int 2011;32:1023–31.
16. Knupp M, Barg A, Bolliger L, et al. Supramalleolar osteotomies for the treatment of overcorrected clubfoot deformity. J Bone Joint Surg Am 2012;94A:1101–7.
17. Hintermann B, Barg A, Knupp M. Corrective supramalleolar osteotomy for malunited pronation-external rotation fractures of the ankle. J Bone Joint Surg Br 2011;93:1367–72.
18. Mann HA, Filippi J, Myerson MS. Intra-articular opening medial tibial wedge osteotomy (plafond-plasty) for the treatment of intra-articular varus ankle arthritis and instability. Foot Ankle Int 2012;33:255–61.
19. Pagenstert GI, Hintermann B, Knupp M. Operative management of chronic ankle instability: plantaris graft. Foot Ankle Clin 2006;11:567–83.
20. Kilger R, Knupp M, Hintermann B. Peroneus longus to peroneus brevis tendon transfer. Techniques in Foot & Ankle Surgery 2009;8:146–9.
21. Stufkens SA, Knupp M, Hintermann B. Medial displacement calcaneal osteotomy. Techniques in Foot & Ankle Surgery 2009;8:85–90.
22. Knupp M, Horisberger M, Hintermann B. A new z-shaped calcaneal osteotomy for 3-plane correction of severe varus deformity of the hindfoot. Techniques in Foot & Ankle Surgery 2008;7:90–5.

23. Tankson CJ. The Cotton osteotomy: indications and techniques. Foot Ankle Clin 2007;12:309–15, vii.
24. Reidsma II, Nolte PA, Marti RK, et al. Treatment of malunited fractures of the ankle: a long-term follow-up of reconstructive surgery. J Bone Joint Surg Br 2010;92:66–70.
25. Hintermann B. Medial ankle instability. Foot Ankle Clin 2003;8:723–38.
26. Hintermann B, Valderrabano V, Kundert HP. Lengthening of the lateral column and reconstruction of the medial soft tissue for treatment of acquired flatfoot deformity associated with insufficiency of the posterior tibial tendon. Foot Ankle Int 1999;20:622–9.
27. Hintermann B, Valderrabano V, Kundert HP. Lateral column lengthening by calcaneal osteotomy combined with soft tissue reconstruction for treatment of severe posterior tibial tendon dysfunction. Methods and preliminary results. Orthopade 1999;28:760–9 [in German].
28. Hintermann B, Renggli P. Anatomic reconstruction of the lateral ligaments of the ankle using a plantaris tendon graft in the treatment of chronic ankle joint instability. Orthopade 1999;28:778–84 [in German].
29. Barg A, Brunner S, Zwicky L, et al. Subtalar and naviculocuneiform fusion for extended breakdown of the medial arch. Foot Ankle Clin 2011;16:69–81.
30. Cheng YM, Huang PJ, Hong SH, et al. Low tibial osteotomy for moderate ankle arthritis. Arch Orthop Trauma Surg 2001;121:355–8.
31. Pagenstert GI, Hintermann B, Barg A, et al. Realignment surgery as alternative treatment of varus and valgus ankle osteoarthritis. Clin Orthop Relat Res 2007; 462:156–68.
32. Takakura Y, Takaoka T, Tanaka Y, et al. Results of opening-wedge osteotomy for the treatment of a post-traumatic varus deformity of the ankle. J Bone Joint Surg Am 1998;80:213–8.
33. Takakura Y, Tanaka Y, Kumai T, et al. Low tibial osteotomy for osteoarthritis of the ankle. Results of a new operation in 18 patients. J Bone Joint Surg Br 1995;77: 50–4.
34. Tanaka Y, Takakura Y, Hayashi K, et al. Low tibial osteotomy for varus-type osteoarthritis of the ankle. J Bone Joint Surg Br 2006;88:909–13.

Is Deltoid and Lateral Ligament Reconstruction Necessary in Varus and Valgus Ankle Osteoarthritis, and How Should These Procedures be Performed?

MaCalus V. Hogan, MD[a],*, David M. Dare, MD[b],
Jonathan T. Deland, MD[c,d],*

KEYWORDS

- Ankle arthritis • Realignment surgery • Valgus ankle deformity
- Deltoid ligament reconstruction • Varus ankle deformity
- Lateral ligament reconstruction

KEY POINTS

- The osseous and soft tissue components of the ankle joint complex work in unison to maintain tibiotalar joint congruency.
- Varus and valgus malalignment of the ankle lead to asymmetric joint wear and degenerative change of the medial and lateral tibiotalar joint, respectively.
- Ligament reconstruction for varus or valgus deformities, when needed, should be performed as an adjunct to bony correction to ensure ligament balance.
- Isolated ligament reconstruction is unlikely to yield acceptable results in the presence of significant osseous deformity or advanced arthritic changes.

Disclosure: None of the authors have received or will receive anything of value from a commercial party/company related directly or indirectly to the subject of this article.
[a] Division of Foot and Ankle Surgery, Department of Orthopaedic Surgery, University of Pittsburgh Medical Center, 5200 Centre Avenue, Pittsburgh, PA 15232, USA; [b] Department of Orthopaedic Surgery, Hospital for Special Surgery, 535 East 70th Street, New York, NY 10021, USA; [c] Division of Foot and Ankle Surgery, Hospital for Special Surgery, 535 East 70th Street, New York, NY 10021, USA; [d] Department of Orthopaedic Surgery, Weill Cornell Medical College, 520 East 70th Street, New York, NY 10021, USA
* Corresponding authors. Division of Foot and Ankle Surgery, Department of Orthopaedic Surgery, University of Pittsburgh Medical Center, 5200 Centre Avenue, Pittsburgh, PA 15232; Division of Foot and Ankle Surgery, Hospital for Special Surgery, 535 East 70th Street, New York, NY 10021.
E-mail addresses: macalushogan@gmail.com; delandj@hss.edu

INTRODUCTION

Varus and valgus ankle deformities represent a challenge to the most experienced foot and ankle surgeons. The presence of degenerative changes of the tibiotalar joint articular surfaces introduces an additional layer of complexity. Reconstruction of such deformities requires a customized approach to each patient. Surgical intervention often calls for joint-sparing realignment, arthroplasty, and/or arthrodesis, depending on the severity of deformity and the joint surface integrity. The ligamentous stability of the ankle plays an essential role in the preservation and optimization of function. This article reviews the role of deltoid and lateral ligament reconstruction in the treatment of varus and valgus ankle osteoarthritis.

CLINICAL EVALUATION

The foot and ankle examination should begin with a carefully obtained history, followed by inspection, palpation, movement, neurovascular examination, and various tests specific to the condition. First, the limb should be exposed to the level of the waist, and overall limb alignment and weight-bearing posture must be assessed while walking and standing. Gait assessment may reveal subtle deformities and loading patterns. Hindfoot and forefoot positions are observed with weight bearing.

Once seated, the examiner may appreciate callus formation in areas of load. It is important to assess the position of the forefoot relative to the hindfoot and declare the relationship supple or rigid. Visualization of the transmalleolar axis aids in determining whether the deformity exists above or below the ankle. Irrespective of the deformity, patients often present with pain. Identifying precise locations of tenderness correlates an anatomic site with a particular disorder. Varus and valgus ankle deformities are associated with particular patterns and locations of pain. The many joints in the foot and ankle should be examined in their primary planes of motion: the ankle in plantar and dorsiflexion, and the subtalar joint in its modified coronal plane. In short, each joint should be assessed individually and all joint lines palpated.

It is crucial that the function and strength of all muscle groups are documented. This requirement is particularly important before consideration of muscle transfers. In this case, all individual muscle agonists and antagonists must be examined to ensure recognition of all deforming forces.[1]

The Achilles tendon must be tested for tightness with the knee both flexed and extended. Restricted dorsiflexion in both positions may represent a contracted posterior capsule or anterior osteophytes. Increased dorsiflexion with the knee flexed indicates a tight gastrocnemius.

The valgus hindfoot has many possible origins. A detailed history and physical examination should aid in elucidating the deformity's cause. With the patient standing, evaluation of the valgus hindfoot reveals a prominent and rounded medial border, in addition to a short, concave lateral border. There may be collapse of the medial longitudinal arch. Hindfoot valgus is best viewed from behind the patient, whereas midfoot abduction should be viewed form a frontal standing view. From this position, the too-many-toes signs and medial-sided swelling are evident.[2]

Next, assess hindfoot biomechanics and flexibility with the double-limb rise. First, note whether the patient can complete the test. Second, note whether the hindfoot inverts with heel rise. Double-limb heel rise should be followed by single-limb heel rise, again noting whether the patient can perform the test and whether the heel inverts.

Hintermann and Gachter[3] initially described the first metatarsal sign. With the patient standing, the shank of the affected foot is externally rotated or the heel is passively aligned into varus. The first metatarsal head elevates in the presence of a dysfunctional posterior tibial tendon and remains on the floor if normal.

With the patient seated, the foot is assessed for medial-sided tenderness and swelling along the course of the posterior tibial tendon (PTT). Lateral-sided tenderness may represent calcaneofibular or sinus tarsi impingement, or subtalar arthritis. When evaluating the strength of the PTT, it must be distinguished from other compensating muscles. Inversion should be tested from a starting position of foot plantarflexion and eversion. This position neutralizes the tibialis anterior.[4] While testing muscle strength, it is crucial to palpate the PTT. It is important to distinguish the presence or absence of PTT contraction in identifying the cause of a valgus hindfoot.

The mobility of the midfoot and hindfoot joints should be determined and any deformity should be labeled mobile or fixed. Joint hypermobility, particularly at the first metatarsal, may be present in the valgus hindfoot. With the lesser metatarsal heads stabilized in maximum dorsiflexion, elevation of the first metatarsal head greater than 8 mm dorsal to the second and third metatarsal heads constitutes hypermobility.[5]

As mentioned earlier, the examiner must appreciate the relationship of the forefoot to the hindfoot. In the valgus hindfoot, the forefoot becomes progressively supinated, such that the foot remains plantigrade. With time, the deformity becomes fixed. With time, the talonavicular, subtalar, and calcaneocuboid joints become fixed and cannot be passively inverted beyond neutral.[6]

Consistent with any examination of the foot and ankle, evaluation for equinus contracture should be included. Distinguishing a tight gastrocnemius from a tight combined gastrocnemius-soleus complex may affect the treatment plan. A similar examination must be performed in evaluation of the varus ankle.

The varus ankle also has many possible causes, likely multifactorial. Inspection should show a varus hindfoot and the presence or absence of claw toes. With the feet aligned straight, the peek-a-boo heel sign may even reveal subtle varus deformities. Inspect for callus formation along the lateral border of the foot, the first metatarsal head, and lateral metatarsal heads. Forefoot varus is seen in clubfoot, after talar neck fracture, or in ankle deformity. Forefoot valgus occurs more frequently with neurologic disorders. The relationship of the forefoot to the hindfoot can be described as supple or rigid.

Ankle palpation may show medial joint line tenderness or anteromedial joint impingement in cases of medial compartment overload. Lateral-sided tenderness represents attenuation of the anterior talofibular ligament (ATFL), calcaneofibular ligament (CFL), or peroneal tendons. Metatarsal head pain identifies the metatarsals carrying additional load. Tenderness to palpation over the second, fourth, or fifth metatarsal shafts may represent a stress fracture.

Passive and active motion should be tested for restrictions in motion, supple or rigid deformities, pain, and crepitus. Assessment of motion in the varus ankle must include passive eversion and inversion, with strength of eversion tested in particular. Excessive talar tilt in neutral represents lateral ligamentous injury. More specifically, the integrity of the ATFL and CFL are tested with the foot in plantarflexion and neutral dorsiflexion, respectively. The anterior drawer test is performed in slight plantarflexion to test for anterior laxity.

Examination of the varus ankle should include the Coleman block test and evaluation for peroneus longus overdrive. The Coleman block test determines whether the hindfoot deformity is correctable. Peroneus longus overdrive, as revealed by excessive plantarflexion of the first metatarsal head, contributes to a varus hindfoot.

PATHOGENESIS OF ANKLE OSTEOARTHRITIS
Varus Deformity

Hindfoot deformities lead to asymmetric force distributions across the joints. Varus hindfoot alignment is the most common alignment in ankle osteoarthritis.[7] The varus hindfoot predisposes to medial joint overload, potentially increasing the rate of cartilage degeneration.[8] In addition to medial joint overload, the varus hindfoot medializes the Achilles pulling vector, thereby generating an inversion moment at the ankle. This inversion moment produces more strain on the lateral ligaments, increasing the potential for lateral instability. Chronic lateral ligament instability is one of the most common causes of ankle osteoarthritis.[9]

Although hip and knee arthritis is predominantly degenerative in nature, most ankle arthritis is posttraumatic in origin. Valderrabano and colleagues[10] reported that 13% of all posttraumatic arthritis cases are caused by a ligamentous lesion, and 85% of these lesions occur in the lateral ligament complex. Persistent ankle instability develops in roughly 20% of those with complete tears.[11] Lateral ligament instability of the ankle causes a deviation of the vertical instant centers of rotation medially, thereby increasing the load on the medial weight-bearing surfaces of the joint, including the medial aspect of the talus and the medial tibial plafond (**Fig. 1**).[12] Harrington[9] reported that narrowing of the medial joint space further medializes vertical instant centers of

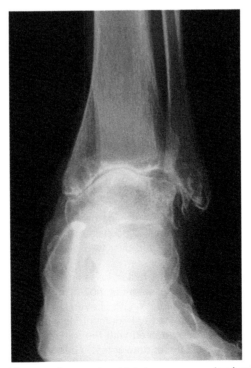

Fig. 1. This patient with varus alignment and joint space narrowing has bony erosion within the ankle. Although lateral ligament reconstruction and bony realignment could be helpful in patients with varus deformity and ankle arthritis, because of the bony erosion and severe joint space narrowing in this case, such a surgery would have a high failure rate. A suitable candidate would be a patient with some joint space remaining, minimal bony erosion, and deformity correctable on a valgus stress view.

rotation and accelerates the arthritic process. In a three-dimensional model of the human ankle, Noguchi[13] found increased contact pressures on the medial side of the ankle after release of the lateral ligaments. Many similar reports have supported this finding.[10,14]

Hashimoto and Inokuchi[15] provided a possible biomechanical explanation for the correlation of lateral ankle instability with ankle osteoarthritis. Patients with a lateral ligament injury abnormally pronate and externally rotate during heel strike, and abnormally supinate and internally rotate during acceleration. The end result is a series of chronic changes in ankle mechanics that may lead to repetitive chondral damage on the medial ankle.

Patients with a severe ankle sprain develop symptomatic end-stage osteoarthritis at a faster rate than patients with recurrent instability.[10] It is speculated that the rate of development of ankle arthritis is associated with the degree of chondral damage at the time of the initial injury. Taga and colleagues[16] were the first to highlight, with the use of arthroscopy, the high incidence of chondral lesions in ankles with recurrent lateral instability. More recently, arthroscopic evaluation detected chondral lesions of the ankle in 77% of patients with recurrent lateral instability. Most of those lesions were located in the medial half of the ankle. These investigators hypothesized that the chondral lesions were a combination of acute chondral injuries and subsequent degenerative changes. Sugimoto and colleagues[17] concluded that, although prolonged instability does not always lead to osteoarthritis, increased patient age, the talar tilt angle, and varus inclination of the plafond were all related to the severity of the chondral lesions, and thus to the development of ankle arthritis.

Valgus Deformity

Valgus alignment is less commonly seen as a cause of ankle osteoarthritis, with studies estimating that it represents 8% to 13% of deformities.[7,18] Several causes of valgus ankle arthritis have been highlighted in the literature. These causes include, but are not limited to, distal tibia and/or fibula malunion, PTT insufficiency, heel cord contracture, posttraumatic arthritis, and deltoid ligament insufficiency (ie, medial ankle ligament instability).[19,20] This article focuses on the role of deltoid ligament injury and insufficiency in the development of valgus ankle osteoarthritis.

The deltoid ligament complex plays an essential role in medial stability to the ankle. It works with adjacent medial ligamentous structures and the distal fibula to prevent talar lateral translation and valgus angulation.[21] The deltoid ligament, also referred to as the medial collateral ligament, is made up of 2 layers (superficial and deep).[22] Injury to the deltoid complex can progress into medial ligamentous instability. In a cadaveric model, Clarke and colleagues[23] showed that deltoid ligament sectioning created a 15% to 20% decrease in ankle joint contract area. Contact area change was irrespective of fibular displacement, with isolated lateral malleolar fracture not causing ankle instability. Injury to the deep deltoid ligament has a higher propensity to lead to lateral and anterior talar translation, as shown in the anatomic sectioning study by Harper.[24] In the same study, superficial deltoid sectioning did not lead to increased talar displacement.[24] The studies discussed earlier highlight the importance of both components of the deltoid complex.[10] Michelson and colleagues,[25] in their cadaveric study, showed that superficial or deep deltoid ligament resulted in significantly increased talar eversion, although only deep deltoid ligament injury led to increased talar internal rotation.

Deltoid ligament insufficiency and associated medial ankle instability are a part of the sequelae of valgus ankle–driven osteoarthritis.[26] Acute injury mechanisms secondary to ankle sprains or fractures, with or without associated ankle disloca-tions, have been shown to encompass deltoid ligament injury.[27] Eversion and external rotation of the ankle strains the deltoid complex. In the setting of supination external rotation (SER) IV, and pronation external rotation (PER) III/IV fractures, the deltoid ligament complex is often disrupted.[28] Although studies have shown that direct deltoid ligament repair is not always necessary in these injury patterns, it remains critical to understand the effects that deltoid incompetence may have on long-term ankle stability.[24,29]

A common chronic cause of deltoid insufficiency is associated with late-stage adult-acquired flatfoot deformity.[21] As a consequence of chronic PTT dysfunction and heel valgus, the deltoid ligament and capsular structures become incompetent. The long-standing medial longitudinal arch collapse and lateralized hindfoot position eventually lead to deltoid ligament dysfunction, resulting in valgus talar tilt (**Fig. 2**).[30] The medial ankle instability and lateral tibiotalar articulation overload over time may lead to artic-ular cartilage degenerative change.[19]

TREATMENT OPTIONS IN VARUS AND VALGUS ANKLE OSTEOARTHRITIS
Conservative Treatment

In cases of arthritic varus or valgus ankles, an attempt at conservative management is warranted. The use of pharmacotherapy with nonsteroidal antiinflammatory medica-tions, custom orthosis, and shoe modifications may yield acceptable results for those with mild deformities.[20] It is essential that these patients are followed clinically to monitor for signs of deformity progression and continuous degenerative change. It is recommended that the treatment algorithm for patients with either varus or valgus deformities be individualized to address all concomitant disorders, to optimize patient outcomes.[19,20]

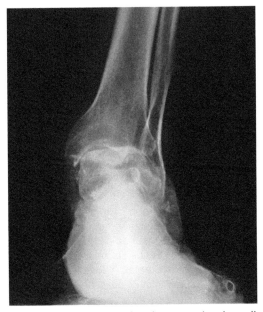

Fig. 2. This patient with valgus deformity has bone erosion laterally. Deltoid ligament reconstruction, even with other bony procedures (except for total ankle or ankle fusion) would not be helpful. This patient underwent total ankle replacement.

Lateral Ligament Reconstruction for Varus Ankle Osteoarthritis

More than 80 surgical procedures have been described as treatment of chronic lateral instability.[31] The many procedures available for chronic lateral instability can be divided into nonanatomic and anatomic reconstructions. In anatomic reconstruction, the natural ligamentous insertions and origins are restored using either endogenous tissue, synthetic graft, or by direct repair. In contrast, nonanatomic reconstruction usually requires use of one of the peroneal tendons, typically that of the peroneal brevis, to regain lateral ankle stability.

Numerous reports have shown restricted ankle range of motion and an absence of normal hindfoot mechanics after nonanatomic repair.[32–34] In addition, nonanatomic reconstruction is associated with a higher rate of complications, including delayed wound healing and nerve injury.[35] In contrast, anatomic reconstruction does not cause restriction of movement and has the potential to restore hindfoot kinematics. As suggested by Schmidt and colleagues,[36] a direct repair of the ligaments should be performed if adequate ligament tissue is present. If not present, the author recommends reconstruction with autograft or allograft tissue passed through drill holes at the insertion points of the ATFL and CFL.

Harrington[9] proposed that lateral ligament reconstruction bears the potential to prevent further degenerative changes, in addition to possibly reversing changes already present, in patients with early signs of medial joint wear. Takao and colleagues[37] recommend lateral ligament reconstruction with arthroscopic drilling for the treatment of stage 2 osteoarthritis. They could not make a similar recommendation for stage 3 osteoarthritis. The ideal candidate for lateral ligament reconstruction in isolation has mild to moderate instability without deformity and possesses viable ligament tissue, absence of hyperlaxity, and a normal body mass index.[38]

The correlation between cavovarus foot deformity and chronic lateral ankle instability is well established. For this reason, Fortin and colleagues[39] propose that lateral ligament reconstruction alone in patients with mild or intermediate arthritis is not sufficient to balance the foot and normalize contact stresses acting across the ankle joint. These patients might not require lateral ligament reconstruction. Sammarco and Taylor[40] reported good to excellent results in patients treated for cavovarus foot without addressing the lateral ligaments. In contrast, Fortin and colleagues[39] noted improved pain and stability in patients treated with lateral ligament reconstruction combined with foot deformity correction. Despite reports by Harrington[9] and Takao and colleagues,[37] there have been no definitive longitudinal studies that assess the efficacy of isolated lateral ligament repair or reconstruction in the treatment of the varus arthritic ankle.

Deltoid Ligament Reconstruction for Valgus Ankle Osteoarthritis

Several techniques for deltoid ligament reconstruction have been described in the literature. Wiltberger and Mallory described a technique using a split PTT autograft. The PTT was left attached to its insertion and the split proximal end of the tendon passed through a bone tunnel in the medial malleolus.[21]

The senior author previously reported a series of 5 patients who underwent stage IV PTT reconstruction along with deltoid reconstruction using peroneus longus tendon autograft. The autograft was passed proximally lateral to medial through the talus, and subsequently medial to lateral from the medial malleolus to the lateral tibia. At a minimum of 2-year follow-up all patients had maintained their respective talar tilt corrections.[26] Furthermore, an intermediate follow-up study of these patients showed that correction and function were maintained.[30]

Jeng and colleagues[41] reported their results of a minimally invasive deltoid ligament reconstruction for patients with stage IV flatfoot deformity. All patients underwent triple arthrodesis combined with deltoid ligament reconstruction using allograft. Five patients were available for final follow-up at a minimum of 20 months. All five were ruled to have had a successful outcome. Tibiotalar valgus decreased from $6.4° \pm 2.9°$ to $2.0° \pm 2.0°$, and lateral tibiotalar joint space was maintained compared with preoperative levels. Functional scores were equal to age-matched normative values as well.

An anatomic reconstructive technique was described by Haddad and colleagues.[42] As originally described, tunnels are created in the distal tibia (deltoid origin), and through the talus and calcaneus for the deep and superficial insertions of the deltoid, respectively. Autograft or allograft tendon can be used. Endobuttons are weaved into each end of the graft, with graft ends passed through the talus and calcaneus respectively. The graft loop is then passed proximally through the drill hole on the tibia and secured to the anterior distal tibia via a cancellous screw and washer construct. The investigators showed that this reconstructive approach recreated eversion and external rotation stability to the talus similar to that achieved by the intact deltoid ligament. It is the senior author's preference to use the technique described by Haddad and colleagues[42] using Achilles allograft, with minor modification, when deltoid reconstruction is needed as an adjunct to comprehensive reconstructive procedures (ie, total ankle arthroplasty, triple arthrodesis, stage IV flatfoot reconstruction) to facilitate medial ligament and tibiotalar joint stability.

Reconstruction of the chronically insufficient deltoid ligament complex can play a role in the treatment algorithm of valgus ankle osteoarthritis, as described by Pagenstert and colleagues.[43] Because most valgus osteoarthritis deformities present in combination with long-standing osseous abnormalities, isolated deltoid soft tissue repair or reconstruction has a low probability of success and is therefore not recommended. Furthermore, we could not identify any support in the literature for isolated deltoid reconstruction for valgus deformity treatment in the setting of arthritic changes of the tibiotalar joint. Consistent with the literature and his experience, the senior author recommends osseous correction in the setting of valgus deformities, with deltoid reconstruction as adjunct when additional ligamentous stability and balancing is needed. In the presence of advanced lateral tibiotalar joint degenerative changes, deltoid ligament reconstruction has therefore not been shown to provide a clinical benefit.

SUMMARY

Varus and valgus ankle deformities represent a challenge to the most experienced foot and ankle surgeons. The presence of degenerative changes of the tibiotalar joint articular surfaces introduces an additional layer of complexity. The ligamentous stability of the ankle plays an essential role in the preservation and optimization of function following surgical reconstruction. Varus and valgus ankle osteoarthritis often present as the later stage of a continuum rooted in both long-standing osseous deformity and soft tissue insufficiency. There is some evidence in the literature that lateral ligament reconstruction, alone, in the setting of progressive medial ankle joint arthritis leads to long-term resolution of patient symptoms and improved outcomes if used as an adjunct to bony correction. We could not identify any evidence supporting isolated deltoid reconstruction for the treatment of valgus osteoarthritis. Deltoid reconstruction is combined with other procedures for stage IV PTT insufficiency in the setting of minimal arthritic change and when lateral joint space is remaining. Our findings are consistent with the senior author's experience.

REFERENCES

1. Thevendran G, Younger AS. Examination of the varus ankle, foot, and tibia. Foot Ankle Clin 2012;17(1):13–20.
2. Johnson KA. Tibialis posterior tendon rupture. Clin Orthop Relat Res 1983;(177): 140–7.
3. Hintermann B, Gachter A. The first metatarsal rise sign: a simple, sensitive sign of tibialis posterior tendon dysfunction. Foot Ankle Int 1996;17(4):236–41.
4. Meehan RE, Brage M. Adult acquired flat foot deformity: clinical and radiographic examination. Foot Ankle Clin 2003;8(3):431–52.
5. Mann RA. Acquired flatfoot in adults. Clin Orthop Relat Res 1983;(181):46–51.
6. Deland JT. Adult-acquired flatfoot deformity. J Am Acad Orthop Surg 2008;16(7): 399–406.
7. Valderrabano V, Horisberger M, Russell I, et al. Etiology of ankle osteoarthritis. Clin Orthop Relat Res 2009;467(7):1800–6.
8. Tarr RR, Resnick CT, Wagner KS, et al. Changes in tibiotalar joint contact areas following experimentally induced tibial angular deformities. Clin Orthop Relat Res 1985;(199):72–80.
9. Harrington KD. Degenerative arthritis of the ankle secondary to long-standing lateral ligament instability. J Bone Joint Surg Am 1979;61(3):354–61.
10. Valderrabano V, Hintermann B, Horisberger M, et al. Ligamentous posttraumatic ankle osteoarthritis. Am J Sports Med 2006;34(4):612–20.
11. Kannus P, Renstrom P. Treatment for acute tears of the lateral ligaments of the ankle. Operation, cast, or early controlled mobilization. J Bone Joint Surg Am 1991;73(2):305–12.
12. Parlasca R, Shoji H, D'Ambrosia RD. Effects of ligamentous injury on ankle and subtalar joints: a kinematic study. Clin Orthop Relat Res 1979;(140):266–72.
13. Noguchi K. Biomechanical analysis for osteoarthritis of the ankle. Nihon Seikei-geka Gakkai Zasshi 1985;59(2):215–22.
14. Bonnel F, Toullec F, Mabit C, et al. Chronic ankle instability: biomechanics and pathomechanics of ligaments injury and associated lesions. Orthop Traumatol Surg Res 2010;96(4):424–32.
15. Hashimoto T, Inokuchi S. A kinematic study of ankle joint instability due to rupture of the lateral ligaments. Foot Ankle Int 1997;18(11):729–34.
16. Taga I, Shino K, Inoue M, et al. Articular cartilage lesions in ankles with lateral ligament injury. An arthroscopic study. Am J Sports Med 1993;21(1):120–6 [discussion: 126–7].
17. Sugimoto K, Takakura Y, Okahashi K, et al. Chondral injuries of the ankle with recurrent lateral instability: an arthroscopic study. J Bone Joint Surg Am 2009; 91(1):99–106.
18. Chou LB, Coughlin MT, Hansen S Jr, et al. Osteoarthritis of the ankle: the role of arthroplasty. J Am Acad Orthop Surg 2008;16(5):249–59.
19. Barg A, Pagenstert GI, Leumann AG, et al. Treatment of the arthritic valgus ankle. Foot Ankle Clin 2012;17(4):647–63.
20. Bluman EM, Chiodo CP. Valgus ankle deformity and arthritis. Foot Ankle Clin 2008;13(3):443–70, ix.
21. Savage-Elliott I, Murawski CD, Smyth NA, et al. The deltoid ligament: an in-depth review of anatomy, function, and treatment strategies. Knee Surg Sports Traumatol Arthrosc 2013;21(6):1316–27.
22. Boss AP, Hintermann B. Anatomical study of the medial ankle ligament complex. Foot Ankle Int 2002;23(6):547–53.

23. Clarke HJ, Michelson JD, Cox QG, et al. Tibio-talar stability in bimalleolar ankle fractures: a dynamic in vitro contact area study. Foot Ankle 1991;11(4):222–7.
24. Harper MC. Deltoid ligament: an anatomical evaluation of function. Foot Ankle 1987;8(1):19–22.
25. Michelson JD, Hamel AJ, Buczek FL, et al. Kinematic behavior of the ankle following malleolar fracture repair in a high-fidelity cadaver model. J Bone Joint Surg Am 2002;84(11):2029 38.
26. Deland JT, de Asla RJ, Segal A. Reconstruction of the chronically failed deltoid ligament: a new technique. Foot Ankle Int 2004;25(11):795–9.
27. Ferran NA, Oliva F, Maffulli N. Ankle instability. Sports Med Arthrosc 2009;17(2):139–45.
28. Schuberth JM, Collman DR, Rush SM, et al. Deltoid ligament integrity in lateral malleolar fractures: a comparative analysis of arthroscopic and radiographic assessments. J Foot Ankle Surg 2004;43(1):20–9.
29. de Souza LJ, Gustilo RB, Meyer TJ. Results of operative treatment of displaced external rotation-abduction fractures of the ankle. J Bone Joint Surg Am 1985;67(7):1066–74.
30. Ellis SJ, Williams BR, Wagshul AD, et al. Deltoid ligament reconstruction with peroneus longus autograft in flatfoot deformity. Foot Ankle Int 2010;31(9):781–9.
31. Muijs SP, Dijkstra PD, Bos CF. Clinical outcome after anatomical reconstruction of the lateral ankle ligaments using the Duquennoy technique in chronic lateral instability of the ankle: a long-term follow-up study. J Bone Joint Surg Br 2008;90(1):50–6.
32. Chrisman OD, Snook GA. Reconstruction of lateral ligament tears of the ankle. An experimental study and clinical evaluation of seven patients treated by a new modification of the Elmslie procedure. J Bone Joint Surg Am 1969;51(5):904–12.
33. Krips R, van Dijk CN, Halasi PT, et al. Long-term outcome of anatomical reconstruction versus tenodesis for the treatment of chronic anterolateral instability of the ankle joint: a multicenter study. Foot Ankle Int 2001;22(5):415–21.
34. Thermann H, Zwipp H, Tscherne H. Treatment algorithm of chronic ankle and subtalar instability. Foot Ankle Int 1997;18(3):163–9.
35. Sammarco VJ. Complications of lateral ankle ligament reconstruction. Clin Orthop Relat Res 2001;(391):123–32.
36. Schmidt R, Cordier E, Bertsch C, et al. Reconstruction of the lateral ligaments: do the anatomical procedures restore physiologic ankle kinematics? Foot Ankle Int 2004;25(1):31–6.
37. Takao M, Komatsu F, Naito K, et al. Reconstruction of lateral ligament with arthroscopic drilling for treatment of early-stage osteoarthritis in unstable ankles. Arthroscopy 2006;22(10):1119–25.
38. Klammer G, Benninger E, Espinosa N. The varus ankle and instability. Foot Ankle Clin 2012;17(1):57–82.
39. Fortin PT, Guettler J, Manoli A 2nd. Idiopathic cavovarus and lateral ankle instability: recognition and treatment implications relating to ankle arthritis. Foot Ankle Int 2002;23(11):1031–7.
40. Sammarco GJ, Taylor R. Cavovarus foot treated with combined calcaneus and metatarsal osteotomies. Foot Ankle Int 2001;22(1):19–30.
41. Jeng CL, Bluman EM, Myerson MS. Minimally invasive deltoid ligament reconstruction for stage IV flatfoot deformity. Foot Ankle Int 2011;32(1):21–30.

42. Haddad SL, Dedhia S, Ren Y, et al. Deltoid ligament reconstruction: a novel technique with biomechanical analysis. Foot Ankle Int 2010;31(7):639–51.
43. Pagenstert GI, Hintermann B, Barg A, et al. Realignment surgery as alternative treatment of varus and valgus ankle osteoarthritis. Clin Orthop Relat Res 2007; 462:156–68.

The Use of Allograft in Joint-preserving Surgery for Ankle Osteochondral Lesions and Osteoarthritis

Brian S. Winters, MD[a], Steven M. Raikin, MD[b],*

KEYWORDS

- Osteochondral lesion of the talus (OLT) • Hemitalectomy
- Fresh osteochondral allograft • Bipolar osteochondral allograft arthroplasty

KEY POINTS

- Large cystic osteochondral lesions of the talus can be salvaged with allograft hemiarthroplasty.
- Fresh osteochondral allografts should be implanted as early as available and within a maximum of 28 days from harvest.
- Fresh Allograft hemiarthroplasty demonstrates better results than allograft total joint bipolar arthroplasty.
- Accuracy of implantation is essential in order to obtain good long term results of osteochondral arthroplasty of the ankle.
- Failure of allograft arthroplasty can be salvaged with an ankle fusion.

INTRODUCTION

Within the foot and ankle, the talar dome is the most common area to develop an osteochondral lesion, termed an osteochondral lesion of the talus (OLT). This is a well-recognized source of ankle pain and dysfunction, most frequently in the young patient, which persists secondary to a limited intrinsic healing potential.[1,2] Patients tend to have a history of trauma to the talus; however, these lesions are also thought to represent an overlap with some degree of osteonecrosis.[3–6] The remaining articular cartilage and the cartilage on the opposing tibial plafond tend to remain well

The authors have no financial disclosures or conflicts of interest related to this topic.
[a] Department of Orthopaedic Surgery, Rothman Institute of Orthopaedics at Thomas Jefferson University Hospital, 1015 Walnut Street, Suite 801, Philadelphia, PA 19107, USA; [b] Department of Orthopaedic Surgery, Rothman Institute of Orthopedics at Thomas Jefferson University Hospital, 925 Chestnut Street, Philadelphia, PA 19107, USA
* Corresponding author.
E-mail address: steven.raikin@rothmaninstitute.com

preserved, as does the joint's range of motion.[1,2] Mixed outcomes in surgical management have been noted because of the unpredictability of cartilage restoration, especially for larger lesions.[7] Potential options for repair or reconstruction include procedures such as arthroscopic debridement combined with microfracture and/or drilling, autologous chondrocyte implantation, and the osteochondral autograft transplant system (OATS)/mosaicplasty.[8–10] However, each of these has limitations in the treatment of large lesions for which the success rates are poor and tissue available for harvest and implantation is limited by risk of harvest site morbidity.

On a similar note, end-stage osteoarthritis of the tibiotalar joint in the young patient, whether posttraumatic in nature or, less often, caused by a large OLT, also presents significant challenges. The gold standard in surgical management has historically been an arthrodesis of the ankle joint, but there has been an increasing desire to preserve ankle joint motion. This desire is a result of long-term deficits noted in gait patterns and the development of adjacent joint degenerative disease, as shown in the arthrodesis literature.[11] For this reason, orthopedic surgeons have searched for practical alternatives in these situations. The most popular currently include the total ankle arthroplasty, supramalleolar osteotomy, and the distraction arthroplasty. These options also have implications when used in the younger patient.

Fresh osteochondral allograft can offer numerous advantages in both of these challenging situations by allowing defective tissue to be anatomically matched and reconstructed through transplantation. The talus in particular is a unique structure, which makes it difficult to match the contours of a graft harvested from, for instance, the femoral condyle to a defect on the talar dome.[12] This difficulty becomes evident especially when treating larger type V and VI lesions, for which multiple OATS plugs may need to be used or a hemitalectomy performed.[1,2,12] There is a quantitative limit as to how much graft can be harvested from the femoral condyle before knee mechanics are altered and the development of arthritis is promoted.[12–14] On a similar note, the bipolar, fresh osteochondral allograft ankle arthroplasty has been sporadically reported in the literature as a potential alternative to ankle fusion in treating end-stage ankle arthritis of young patients. The theoretic advantage of this approach is that the ankle is biologically resurfaced in order to preserve motion.

Fresh osteochondral allografts provide a means to transplant mature hyaline cartilage, with viable chondrocytes that can sustain its surrounding collagen matrix, into a large defect in order to recreate a congruent joint.[1,2,7,10,15,16] Understanding the processes of tissue recovery, different storage methods, safety concerns, sterilization procedures, and the immunologic ramifications is a vital first step in achieving a successful outcome.

BASIC SCIENCE

Fresh osteochondral transplants were initially performed in the knee for large focal defects and osteoarthritis. They did not become popularized for use in the ankle joint for many years and therefore most of the basic science literature comes from experiences in the knee. Several things should be considered when the decision is made to use fresh osteochondral allograft tissue.

The American Association of Tissue Banks (AATB) was established to help ensure that donor tissue is handled appropriately.[17] Of the approximately 1300 tissue banks located throughout the United States, only 100 are accredited by the AATB, of which 88 distribute musculoskeletal tissues. Despite this, approximately 10% of allografts currently used in orthopedic surgery still originate from a nonaccredited tissue bank.[18,19] It is therefore especially important to know who the supplier is otherwise clinicians may increase their chances of failure.[17,20,21] Tissue-banking standards and quality control protocols are important and must be strictly followed in order to increase the likelihood of obtaining an acceptable graft. Once the graft has cleared all checkpoints, the specimen is ready for processing.[18,19]

Osteochondral allograft tissue is prepared and stored in 3 different forms in the United States and each has its advantages and disadvantages. They include freeze dried; fresh frozen; and fresh, cold-stored. This article concentrates on fresh cold-stored tissue, because it is the optimal tissue to use for transplantation when treating the large OLT and end-stage ankle arthritis.

The tissue is harvested soon after donor demise and stored refrigerated at 4°C. With this method, studies have shown that 97% of chondrocytes remain viable for up to 14 days following harvest but viability decreases with time, and only 70% viability is evident by day 28.[10] Mechanical properties are also well maintained within this time frame. No significant differences were noted in glycosaminoglycan content, indentation stiffness, compressive modulus, permeability, or tensile modulus compared with initial values.[10] Specimens stored longer than 28 days began to undergo a significant decrease in metabolic activity with resultant matrix degradation and therefore should not be used.[7,10,16] As a result, the use of fresh cold-stored tissue implanted close to 14 days from procurement has been supported.[2,7,10] The optimal method of cold storage has also been a topic of interest. Literature has shown that fetal bovine serum added to the media increases chondrocyte viability and cell density compared with serum-free media.[22] Proteoglycan synthesis in the allograft cartilage (measured by 35-sulfate radioactive tracer incorporation) also increases with the inclusion of fetal bovine serum.[22] In addition, gradual rewarming of the allograft and treatment with nitric oxide synthase inhibitor at the time of transplantation are beneficial in reversing the metabolic suppression that occurs during cold storage.[23]

ALLOGRAFT CONCERNS

When using fresh tissues, the potential for disease transmission remains of major concern. To help avoid this serious complication, the US Food and Drug Administration and the AATB have set forth several guidelines but deficiencies in the process continue to be reported, which results in a large number of musculoskeletal allografts being recalled every year.[24] The guidelines now include obtaining an initial, detailed history of the donor and performing a series of serologic and bacterial tests.[16] Although few have been reported in the literature, there have been instances of bacterial infection after allograft transplantation. However, all of these have occurred with soft tissue (tendon or meniscal) allografts and are thought to be caused by postprocessing contamination.[25–28] In 2002, the Centers for Disease Control and Prevention published their 7-year study, which showed 23 confirmed physician-reported infections, of which 13 were of *Clostridium* species.[29] In 2003 and 2006, there were also reports of a *Streptococcus pyogenes* (group A *Streptococcus*) and *Chryseobacterium meningosepticum* infection, respectively, following knee ligament reconstructive surgery.[24,28,30] A less common occurrence is the contraction of a viral infection. The risk of transmitting the human immunodeficiency virus (HIV) with modern screening techniques is roughly 1 in 1.6 million,[24,31] and only 4 cases of hepatitis have been documented in the literature.[32,33] However, the process of testing for infectious agents takes on average 14 days to receive the results and continues to be the rate-limiting step to transplantation.

Because current practice does not require human leukocyte antigen (HLA) or blood-type matching, the immunologic ramifications of using a fresh osteochondral allograft must also be considered.[16] These grafts continue to elicit a variable immune response despite hyaline cartilage being considered an immune-privileged tissue.[16,34] In one study, 57% of patients receiving a fresh osteochondral allograft generated serum anti-HLA antibodies, signifying immune sensitization.[35] A possible explanation for this result is related to the osseous portion of the graft, which possesses cells expressing HLA that intimately interact with the recipient, although some do not think that these cells survive the transplantation. As shown by a lone case report in the literature of an acute rejection,[36] patients generally tolerate the transplant with little or no histologic evidence of rejection or delayed graft incorporation.[34] Although humoral immunity may play a role in the final outcome, its clinical relevance remains unknown. In addition, there is the theoretic concern of a patient developing a malignancy from an allograft, but this remains theoretic because it has never been documented in the literature.

The final step before transplantation involves tissue sterilization, which is a delicate balance between preserving biological function and removing all microorganisms. The ideal method would eliminate all potential pathogens from the graft without compromising its viability or any of its biomechanical properties. However, no such mechanism exists and all sterilization processes have the potential to affect a graft in an adverse manner. Because all methods are less than ideal, it is necessary to adhere to strict sterile technique during the procurement and storage phases in order to reduce the risk for tissue contamination and cross-contamination.

In the past, gamma irradiation has been the most widely used method for musculoskeletal allografts, with the standard dose being approximately 10 to 15 kGy. This dose minimizes the risk of bacterial transmission to approximately 1 in 1 million and allows the graft to maintain its biomechanical properties.[37] However, the elimination of HIV requires a higher dose of radiation, estimated to be between 30 and 40 kGy,[38] and studies have shown that doses of 30 kGy can significantly alter graft properties, making 25 kGy the current recommended maximal dose.[39] Therefore, HIV cannot be eliminated using this method without jeopardizing graft integrity. Antibiotic soaks are typically used synergistically with this method as well.

REVIEW OF THE LITERATURE
Allograft OATS and Bulk Talus Osteochondral Allografts

For symptomatic, osteochondral lesions measuring up to 1 cm^3 that do not respond to conservative treatment, arthroscopic debridement and microfracture or drilling is widely recognized as the gold standard. However, this results in a fibrocartilaginous tissue filling the defect,[40–42] which has been shown to produce suboptimal results for larger lesions, cystic lesions, and lesions requiring revision.[43–47] In conjunction with the morbidity associated with obtaining autografts, this led to the development of the allograft osteochondral transfer system.

Although the literature on the OATS/mosaicplasty technique is not as extensive as for autograft OATS, the results have been comparable in their success rates. The largest study to date was reported by El-Rahidy and colleagues[48] in 2011 on their series of 38 patients. They used fresh osteochondral allograft as the donor tissue and, at 38 months, saw the average Visual Analog Scale (VAS) and American Orthopaedic Foot and Ankle Society (AOFAS)–Ankle-Hindfoot (AH) scores improve significantly: 8.2 to 3.3 and 52 to 79, respectively. Four patients out of the 38 had a poor outcome (10.5% failure rate), all of whom were noted to have had a prior operation or additional disorder. This finding shows that, when used in the appropriate setting, the allograft OATS technique can recreate a congruent joint and, more importantly, significantly improve patient function and decrease pain.

Most of the literature on allograft osteochondral transfers has been with regard to lesions that require a hemitalectomy with bulk allograft transplantation. This technique has been described for the reconstruction of extensive talar dome involvement or massive type VI OLT (large cystic lesions with volume greater than 3000 mm^3),[1] with success rates ranging between 66% and 100%.[2,49–52] The first series was reported by Gross and colleagues[51] in 2001, but was limited by the lack of any validated outcome scores. However, they did show a 66% survival rate at an average of 11 years after surgery. The remaining 34% ultimately required ankle arthrodesis secondary to graft resorption and fragmentation.

In 2009, Raikin,[2] the senior author of this article published his series of patients with type VI OLT. With an average of 54 months follow-up, he noted an 87% graft survival rate, as well as a high level of patient satisfaction, with 73% reporting good or excellent results. Outcome measures supported this because a significant improvement was seen in the mean VAS (8.5–3.3) and AOFAS-AH (38–83) scores ($P<.05$).

Since this publication, an additional 11 cases (current total of 26 cases) have been performed with a minimum of 12 months follow-up. There have been 18 men and 8 women, with an average age of 40.2 years (range 16–62 years). There were 15 right and 11 left ankles involved, with the medial talus requiring reconstruction in 20 (77%) of the cases. These procedures continue to be performed on large talar lesions with an average size of 5540 cm^2 (range 3003–10,120 cm^2). Sixteen of the patients had undergone at least one prior surgery on their ankles. At an average of 65 months follow-up (range 14–128 months, with 14 patients currently more than 5 years after implantation with surviving allografts), a total of 3 allografts had failed (88.5% survival), which includes the 2 patients who were previously reported as requiring fusion at 32 and 76 months, respectively.

A third and more recent patient was a 51-year-old woman with a massive cystic type VI lesion shown on a preoperative computed tomography (CT) scan (**Fig. 1**). She in turn received a hemitalectomy with bulk talus allograft transplantation and, at her 6-month postoperative visit, reported improvement of her pain and the graft showed good incorporation (**Fig. 2**). However, she began to develop resorption of the allograft starting at 18 months following implantation (**Fig. 3**). The patient subsequently underwent an arthroscopic debridement with screw removal after 25 months (**Fig. 4**) and was converted to a fusion with tricortical iliac crest bone graft augmentation 31 months after implantation (**Fig. 5**).

The remaining patients reported persistent improvement in function with a preoperative average VAS score of 8.65 improving to 2.9 at most recent follow-up. At present, 21 of the surviving 23 patients with allograft hemitalar arthroplasties (80.8% of the 26 implanted) self-rate their results as good or excellent.

In 2010, Hahn and colleagues[52] published a series of 13 patients with an average of 48 months follow-up, which showed significant improvement in Foot Function Index and AOFAS-AH scores from 5.56 to 2.01 ($P<.05$) and 45 to 81 ($P<.05$), respectively. Gortz and colleagues,[50] also in 2010, published an 83% survival rate in 12 ankles (10/12) at 38 months follow-up. Clinical outcome was evaluated by using the Olerud-Molander Ankle Score (OMAS), which showed a mean improvement from 28 to 71 points ($P<.05$), with 30% of patients reporting excellent, 20% good, and 20% poor results. This finding in turn translated into 90% being satisfied, 60% seeing improved function, and 80% having reduced pain.

Adams and colleagues[49] had the most success to date in the literature, as shown by their 2011 report of a 100% survival rate in 8 patients with a mean follow-up of 4 years. Although 5 patients in this series showed radiographic lucencies at the graft-host interface, none warranted a subsequent procedure at the time of publication. There

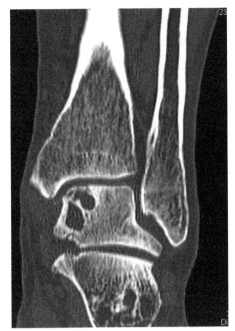

Fig. 1. Coronal cut CT scan showing the large multicystic lesion in the medial talar dome with intra-articular extension and collapse.

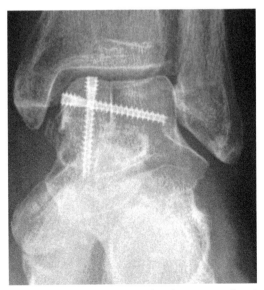

Fig. 2. Anteroposterior (AP) radiograph at 6 months after surgery showing a stable allograft in good position with signs of early osseointegration of the talus allograft.

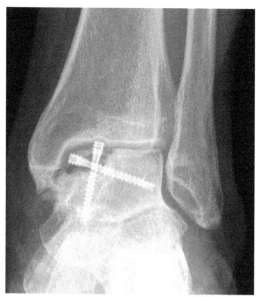

Fig. 3. AP radiograph at 18 months after surgery showing late rejection of the allograft transplant as shown by the resorption with resultant collapse.

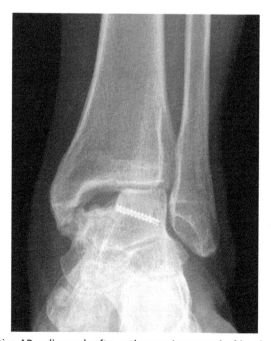

Fig. 4. Postoperative AP radiograph after arthroscopic removal of hardware and allograft resection.

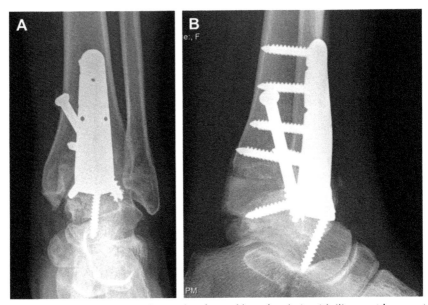

Fig. 5. AP (A) and lateral (B) radiographs after ankle arthrodesis with iliac crest bone autograft augmentation with plate and screw fixation.

was a significant improvement in the mean Lower Extremity Functional Scale score from 37 to 65 points, as well as a reduction in pain with VAS scores reducing from a mean of 6 points to 1 point.

Unlike those previously discussed, Haene and colleagues[53] performed a prospective study in 2012 with 49 months follow-up, which suggested a more guarded conclusion. Seventeen ankles received a fresh osteochondral allograft, of which 16 had at least one prior surgery. With the assistance of plain radiographs and CT scans, failure of graft incorporation with subsequent subsidence was identified in 2 cases. Osteolysis and subchondral cysts were also present in 5 and 8 of the grafts, respectively, whereas there were degenerative changes outside the graft area in 7 ankles. Ankle Osteoarthritis (AOS) Disability and American Academy of Orthopedic Surgeons Foot and Ankle Core Scale scores both significantly improved from 53.4 before surgery to 36.9 after surgery ($P = .03$) and from 52.3 to 69.9 ($P = .02$), respectively. The AOS Pain and Short Form-36 (SF-36) Physical Component Summary scores both showed some improvement; however, they were not statistically significant. There was similarly no significant change in the SF-36 Mental Component Summary and AAOS Foot and Ankle Shoe Comfort Scale scores. Clinical status was ultimately stratified, which showed an excellent or good outcome in 10 ankles (59% success rate) and 5 considered to be failures (29%).

The evidence currently in the literature suggests and reinforces that indications for this procedure need to be carefully evaluated and that the patient should be properly educated before it is considered as a surgical option.

Osteochondral Allograft Ankle Arthroplasty

Long-term results of ankle fusion in young patients have shown high rates of adjacent joint arthritis, pain, and dysfunction. Because of the current limited longevity of ankle arthroplasty systems, metallic joint replacement similarly remains problematic in young patients. As a result, fresh osteochondral allograft replacement has been suggested as an alternative for end-stage arthritis of the ankle in young patients.

Brage and colleagues[54] first reported on the use of osteochondral allograft treatment of ankle cartilage disorders in 2002. Since then, allograft replacement has been studied internationally, but all current published studies have been level 4 or 5 data, retrospective reviews, without control groups, and predominantly retrospectively collected data. Most studies have focused on young patients with an average age of 38.7 years.

The first published results in 2002 by Kim and colleagues[55] from University of California, San Diego (UCSD), reported on 7 patients in a level 4 study. Their technique used freehand saw cuts to resect the arthritic bone and create a matching allograft, performed through an anterior surgical approach. Fixation was obtained with bioabsorbable pins or Herbert screws. At a minimum follow-up period of 7 years (average 148 months), they reported a 42% procedure failure as defined by requiring revision surgery or ankle fusion. The remaining patients whose ankle allografts had survived showed improved functional scores in all parameters measured, but none were statistically significant. As in all subsequent studies, they showed a high percentage of advanced radiographic degenerative changes in surviving ankles, with little correlation between radiographic and final clinical/functional results. They concluded that an imprecise graft fit resulted in poor results.

Based on Kim and colleagues[55] recommendations for more accurate cuts and matching graft fit, Tontz and colleagues[56] described using the Agility total ankle system (DePuy, Warsaw, IN) cutting jigs to improve the accuracy of the allograft fit within the host ankle. Performed at the same UCSD facility as Kim and colleagues[55] cases, they reported that, at the 21-month follow-up, 42% of ankles required additional surgery but only 1 required revision for graft collapse when using the Agility jigs.

In 2005, Meehan and colleagues[57] again reported results from the same institution on 11 patients in whom graft had been cut and fitted using the Agility total ankle arthroplasty system jigs (level 4 study). Five of the 11 (45.5%) cases resulted in failure at average follow-up of 33 months (minimum 24 months). They attributed failure to mismatch of the graft size and thickness of the graft used, with a higher failure rate noted if graft thickness was less than 7 mm. Surviving allografts in their series showed a significant improvement in pain, gait, and function, although most required additional surgical joint debridement or hardware removal. Patients in the study were not HLA matched to donors and 10 out of 11 (91%) showed cytotoxic HLA antibodies in their serum at 6 months. However, there was no correlation between HLA antibody levels and failure of the allograft. Most surviving grafts again showed moderate to advanced degenerative changes radiographically, with little correlation between radiographic and clinical results.

An alternate approach was presented by Vora and Parks[58] in 2005 (Vora and Parks, unpublished data, 2005) in which allografts were implanted via a lateral approach using a curved saw blade resurfacing system. At 1-year follow-up, 50% failure was reported in their 10 patients.

The first published study from an institution other than UCSD was published by Jeng and colleagues[59] from Baltimore, Maryland. Using the Agility jig system, distraction external fixation, and meticulous positioning and bone cuts, 29 fresh allograft were implanted and followed for an average of 24 months (level 4 study). Forty-eight percent of the grafts (14 out of 29) had failed and been revised to total ankle arthroplasties (3); ankle arthrodesis with femoral head allograft interposition (5); repeat osteochondral allograft (5), of which 2 subsequently failed; and 1 fusion using a compressive external fixator and multiple debridements for infection. In addition to the 14 failures, an additional 6 patients had radiographic failures with graft collapse, allograft fracture, or severe joint space narrowing and were pending revision. This outcome resulted in a 31% success rate in their series. They attributed higher failure rates to younger patients (the average age in the success group was 45.7 years compared with 38.4 years in the failure group); high body mass index (24.3 in the success group, 28.4 in the failure group); and persistent deformity following implantation (coronal plane deformity was 2.4° in the success group, 5.8° in the failure group), with the additional suggestion that graft thickness may affect survival of the allograft. There was no correlation between donor age or the time from harvest to implantation and the outcome of the procedure.

A case report was published in 2011 in which the investigators performed a hybrid tibial-sided, fresh osteochondral allograft resurfacing and a talar-sided, fresh osteochondral allograft mosiacplasty.[60] At 66-month follow-up, the final radiograph showed complete integration of the allograft with mild joint space narrowing. The patient also showed no limp with walking and was able to participate in tennis and snow skiing with no pain. Western Ontario and McMaster Universities (WOMAC) Osteoarthritis Index, total WOMAC, and AOFAS-AH scores after surgery supported this observation and were 0, 94, and 98, respectively.

The most recent study published on osteochondral allograft ankle arthroplasty was from the Rizzoli Institute in Bologna, Italy (level 4 study). Giannini and colleagues[61] reported on 32 patients with an average 31-month follow-up (minimum 24 months). As in the study by Vora and Parks,[58] these grafts were inserted via a lateral surgical approach with custom cutting jigs for harvest and implantation. This method may limit the change of incongruence between the graft and host surfaces, whereas the curved tibia cut increases the surface area for allograft fixation and in-growth. The investigators proposed that delayed weight bearing was required to protect the allograft from fracture and collapse. Their patients were kept non–weight bearing for 4 months, followed by an additional 2 months at 30 kg (66 pounds) weight bearing in a fracture boot. The most common complication reported was nonunion of the fibular osteotomy. Only 9 grafts (19%) failed requiring revision, with 53% of patients reporting excellent or good results. Again, all patients had radiographic evidence of advanced degenerative arthritis (grade 2–3 on Van Dijk Arthritis Scale), but no correlation was shown between radiographic findings and clinical outcome. In addition, unlike in the study by Jeng and colleagues,[59] no correlation was found between patient age and their outcomes. The first 7 of their patients underwent cartilage biopsy at 6 months, which showed disorganized collagen, low proteoglycan levels, and increased surface fibrocartilage levels. Patients were not matched for ABO or HLA typing, and all patients tested had evidence of catabolic factors within the biopsied cartilage.

In addition, the same group from the Rizzoli Institute recently published a case report in which they described the taking down of a painful ankle fusion and conversion to a bipolar allograft arthroplasty.[17] This anecdotal report showed a 20° painless arc of motion with a 58-point improvement in AOFAS-AH score after 44 months. This procedure was performed though an anterior approach using a BOX total ankle system cutting jig (Finsbury Orthopaedics, United Kingdom), and not the lateral approach that they describe in the primary technique.

SUMMARY

In conclusion, fresh osteochondral allograft arthroplasty is an option for young patients with advanced arthritic involvement of their ankle joints who have failed nonsurgical interventions, and in whom arthrodesis or metallic arthroplasty is considered a poor option. Optimal host-graft size matching and fit, postimplantation limb alignment, and meticulous implantation technique have been shown to improve outcome. However, there remains a high complication and failure rate of this technically demanding procedure and factors such as the optimal graft thickness, histocompatibility matching, and duration of postimplantation non–weight-bearing status remain unclear.

There are currently few published studies on osteochondral allograft arthroplasty, all of which have level IV evidence with short follow-up. Although in theory this procedure is a potentially desirable option for a young patient with advanced ankle arthritis, it has a high level of technical difficulty and complications with the reported results showing a high failure rate. If this procedure is to be used, it is imperative to educate the patient about the potential consequences and prior published results in order to obtain adequate informed consent.

REFERENCES

1. Raikin S. Stage VI: massive osteochondral defects of the talus. Foot Ankle Clin 2004;9:737–44.
2. Raikin S. Fresh osteochondral allografts for large-volume cystic osteochondral defects of the talus. J Bone Joint Surg Am 2009;91(12):2818–26.
3. Anderson IF, Crichton KJ, Grattan-Smith T, et al. Osteochondral fractures of the dome of the talus. J Bone Joint Surg Am 1989;71(8):1143–52.
4. Barnes CJ, Ferkel RD. Arthroscopic debridement and drilling of osteochondral lesions of the talus. Foot Ankle Clin 2003;8(2):243–57.
5. Berndt AL, Harty M. Transchondral fractures (osteochondritis dissecans) of the talus. J Bone Joint Surg Am 1959;41:988–1020.
6. Canale ST, Belding RH. Osteochondral lesions of the talus. J Bone Joint Surg Am 1980;62(1):97–102.
7. Malinin T, Temple T, Buck B. Transplantation of osteochondral allografts after cold storage. J Bone Joint Surg Am 2006;88(4):762–70.
8. Marcacci M, Kon E, Zaffagnini S, et al. Use of autologous grafts for reconstruction of osteochondral defects of the knee. Orthopedics 1999;22:595–600.
9. Minas T. Autologous chondrocyte implantation for focal chondral defects of the knee. Clin Orthop 2001;(Suppl 391):S349–61.
10. Williams S, Amiel D, Ball S, et al. Prolonged storage effects on the articular cartilage of fresh human osteochondral allografts. J Bone Joint Surg Am 2003; 85(11):2111–20.
11. Coester LM, Saltzman CL, Leupold J, et al. Long-term results following ankle arthrodesis for post-traumatic arthritis. J Bone Joint Surg Am 2001;83:219–28.
12. Marymont JV, Shute G, Zhu H, et al. Computerized matching of autologous femoral grafts for the treatment of medial talar osteochondral defects. Foot Ankle Int 2005;26(9):708–12.
13. Reddy S, Pedowitz DI, Parekh SG, et al. The morbidity associated with osteochondral harvest from asymptomatic knees for the treatment of osteochondral lesions of the talus. Am J Sports Med 2007;35(1):80–5.
14. Valderrabano V, Leumann A, Rasch H, et al. Knee-to-ankle mosaicplasty for the treatment of osteochondral lesions of the ankle joint. Am J Sports Med 2009; 1(Suppl 37):105S–11S.
15. Giannini S, Buda R, Cavallo M, et al. Conversion of painful ankle arthrodesis to bipolar fresh osteochondral allograft: case report. Foot Ankle Int 2012;33(8):678–81.

16. Gortz S, Bugbee W. Allografts in articular cartilage repair. J Bone Joint Surg Am 2006;88(6):1374–84.
17. Rules and Regulations. Federal Register; vol.69, No. 226. Available at: http://www.gpo.gov/fdsys/pkg/FR-2004-11-24/pdf/04-25798.pdf. Accessed November 24, 2004..
18. Jacobs NJ. Establishing a surgical bone bank. In: Fawcett K, Barr A, editors. Tissue banking. Arlington (VA): American Association of Blood Banks; 1987. p. 67–96.
19. Standards for tissue banking. Arlington (VA): American Association of Tissue Banks; 1987.
20. University of Miami Tissue Bank. Available at: http://umiamitb.org.
21. Allosource. Available at: http://www.allosource.org.
22. Pennock AT, Wagner F, Robertson CM, et al. Prolonged storage of osteochondral allografts: does the addition of fetal bovine serum improve chondrocyte viability? J Knee Surg 2006;19:265–72.
23. Pylawka TK, Virdi AS, Cole BJ, et al. Reversal of suppressed metabolism in prolonged cold preserved cartilage. J Orthop Res 2008;26:247–54.
24. Joyce MJ, Greenwald AS, Boden S, et al. Musculoskeletal Allograft Tissue Safety. Presented at the 75th Annual Meeting of the American Academy of Orthopaedic Surgeons, San Francisco, March 5–9th, 2008.
25. Deijkers RL, Bloem RM, Petit PL, et al. Contamination of bone allografts: analysis of incidence and predisposing factors. J Bone Joint Surg Br 1997;79(1):161–6.
26. Kuehnert MJ, Clark E, Lockhart SR, et al. *Candida albicans* endocarditis associated with a contaminated aortic valve allograft: implications for regulation of allograft processing. Clin Infect Dis 1998;27(4):688–91.
27. Malinin TI, Buck BE, Temple HT, et al. Incidence of clostridial contamination in donors' musculoskeletal tissue. J Bone Joint Surg Br 2003;85(7):1051–4.
28. Mroz TE, Joyce MJ, Steinmetz MP, et al. Musculoskeletal allograft risks and recalls in the United States. J Am Acad Orthop Surg 2008;16(10):559–65.
29. Centers for Disease Control and Prevention (CDC). Update: allograft-associated bacterial infections—United States, 2002. MMWR Morb Mortal Wkly Rep 2002; 51(10):207–10.
30. Cartwright EJ, Prabhu RM, Zinderman CE, Food and Drug Administration Tissue Safety Team Investigators. Transmission of *Elizabethkingia meningoseptica* (formerly *Chryseobacterium meningosepticum*) to tissue-allograft recipients: a report of two cases. J Bone Joint Surg Am 2010;92(6):1501–6.
31. Boyce T, Edwards J, Scarborough N. Allograft bone: the influence of processing on safety and performance. Orthop Clin North Am 1999;30(4):571–81.
32. Shutkin NM. Homologous-serum hepatitis following the use of refrigerated bone-bank bone. J Bone Joint Surg Am 1954;36(1):160–2.
33. Tomford WW. Transmission of disease through transplantation of musculoskeletal allografts. J Bone Joint Surg Am 1995;77(11):1742–54.
34. Ward WG, Gautreaux MD, Lippert DC 2nd, et al. HLA sensitization and allograft bone graft incorporation. Clin Orthop Relat Res 2008;466(8):1837–48.
35. Sirlin CB, Brossmann J, Boutin RD, et al. Shell osteochondral allografts of the knee: comparison of MR imaging findings and immunologic responses. Radiology 2001;219:35–43.
36. Hamlet W, Liu SH, Yang R. Destruction of a cryopreserved meniscal allograft: a case for acute rejection. Arthroscopy 1997;13(4):517–21.
37. DeLee JC, Drez D, Miller M. DeLee and Drez's sports medicine: principles and practices. 3rd edition. Philadelphia: Saunders; 2010.

38. Conway B, Tomford W, Mankin HJ, et al. Radiosensitivity of HIV-1: potential application to sterilization of bone allografts. AIDSlink 1991;5:608–9.
39. Paulos LE, France EP, Rosenberg TD, et al. Comparative material properties of allograft tissues for ligament replacement: effects of type, age, sterilization and preservation. Trans Orthop Res Soc 1987;12:129.
40. Kumai T, Takakura Y, Higashiyama I, et al. Arthroscopic drilling for the treatment of osteochondral lesions of the talus. J Bone Joint Surg Am 1999;81(9): 1229–35.
41. Lahm A, Erggelet C, Steinwachs M, et al. Arthroscopic management of osteochondral lesions of the talus: results of drilling and usefulness of magnetic resonance imaging before and after treatment. Arthroscopy 2000;16:299–304.
42. Parisien JS, Vangsness T. Operative arthroscopy of the ankle. Three years' experience. Clin Orthop Relat Res 1985;199:46–53.
43. Becher C, Therman H. Results of microfracture in the treatment of articular cartilage defects of the talus. Foot Ankle Int 2005;26:583–9.
44. Robinson DE, Winson IG, Harries WJ, et al. Arthroscopic treatment of osteochondral lesions of the talus. J Bone Joint Surg Br 2003;85:989–93.
45. Schimmer RC, Dick W, Hintermann B. The role of ankle arthroscopy in the treatment strategies of osteochondritis dissecans lesions of the talus. Foot Ankle Int 2001;22:895–900.
46. Scranton PE Jr, Frey CC, Feder KS. Outcome of osteochondral autograft transplantation for type-V cystic osteochondral lesions of the talus. J Bone Joint Surg Br 2006;88:614–9.
47. Scranton PE Jr, McDermott JE. Treatment of type V osteochondral lesions of the talus with ipsilateral knee osteochondral autografts. Foot Ankle Int 2001;22(5): 380–4.
48. El-Rashidy H, Villacis D, Omar I, et al. Fresh osteochondral allograft for the treatment of cartilage defects of the talus: a retrospective review. J Bone Joint Surg Am 2011;93(17):1634–40.
49. Adams SB Jr, Viens NA, Easley ME, et al. Midterm results of osteochondral lesions of the talar shoulder treated with fresh osteochondral allograft transplantation. J Bone Joint Surg Am 2011;93(7):648–54.
50. Gortz S, De Young AJ, Bugbee WD. Fresh osteochondral allografting for osteochondral lesions of the talus. Foot Ankle Int 2010;31:283–90.
51. Gross AE, Agnidis Z, Hutchison CR. Osteochondral defects of the talus treated with fresh osteochondral allograft transplantation. Foot Ankle Int 2001;22:385–91.
52. Hahn DB, Aanstoos ME, Wilkins RM. Osteochondral lesions of the talus treated with fresh talar allografts. Foot Ankle Int 2010;31:277–82.
53. Haene R, Qamirani E, Story RA, et al. Intermediate outcomes of fresh talar osteochondral allografts for treatment of large osteochondral lesions of the talus. J Bone Joint Surg Am 2012;94(12):1105–10.
54. Brage ME, Bugbee W, Tontz W. Intraoperative and postoperative complications of fresh tibiotalar allografting. Presented at the Annual Winter meeting of the American Orthopaedic Foot and Ankle Society, Dallas, February 13–17, 2002.
55. Kim CW, Jamali A, Tontz W Jr, et al. Treatment of post-traumatic ankle arthrosis with bipolar tibiotalar osteochondral shell allografts. Foot Ankle Int 2002;23(12): 1091–102.
56. Tontz WL Jr, Bugbee WD, Brage ME. Use of allografts in the management of ankle arthritis. Foot Ankle Clin 2003;8(2):361–73, xi.
57. Meehan R, McFarlin S, Bugbee W, et al. Fresh ankle osteochondral allograft transplantation for tibiotalar joint arthritis. Foot Ankle Int 2005;26(10):793–802.

58. Vora A, Parks, B. Early failure of bipolar osteochondral tibiotalar allograft replacements. Presented at the annual winter meeting of the American Orthopaedics Foot and Ankle Society, Washington, DC, February 23–27, 2005.

59. Jeng CL, Kadakia A, White KL, et al. Fresh osteochondral total ankle allograft transplantation for the treatment of ankle arthritis. Foot Ankle Int 2008;29(6): 554–60.

60. Pearsall AW 4th, Madanagopal SG, Jacob J. Modified technique for unipolar allograft ankle replacement: midterm follow-up. A case report. Am J Orthop (Belle Mead NJ) 2011;40(4):E67–70.

61. Giannini S, Buda R, Grigolo B, et al. Bipolar fresh osteochondral allograft of the ankle. Foot Ankle Int 2010;31(1):38–46.

Chondral and Osteochondral Reconstruction of Local Ankle Degeneration

Martin Wiewiorski, MD[a,b,*], Alexej Barg, MD[a],
Victor Valderrabano, MD, PhD[a,*]

KEYWORDS

- Ankle • Cartilage • Osteoarthritis • Osteochondral lesion

KEY POINTS

- Osteochondral lesions of the talus are mostly posttraumatic.
- Surgical treatment techniques can be categorized into non–tissue transplantation and tissue transplantation methods.
- Supplemental procedures to restore alignment and stability are recommended.
- The level of evidence of surgical outcome studies is poor.

LOCAL ANKLE DEGENERATION

The term originally used for this entity was osteochondritis dissecans and was first applied by Kappis in 1922.[1] Other commonly used names are flake fracture, osteochondral fracture, transchondral fracture, or osteochondral defect. Expert consensus and recent literature have coined the term osteochondral lesion of the talus (OCLT) to encompass all previously used terminology (regardless of cause or morphology, and including purely cartilaginous or combined cartilage-bone lesions).[2] Because of the number of varying classifications used in small case series it is hard to determine the proportion of purely cartilaginous lesions (0%–77.5%) to combined osteochondral lesions (12.5%–100%).[3,4] OCLT can be seen as a local degeneration of the ankle joint.

CAUSES OF OCLT

The natural history of OCLT remains unclear, because most patients receive treatment. Daily clinical experience suggesting OCLT to be primarily caused by trauma

Disclosure: The authors have nothing to disclose.
[a] Orthopaedic Department, University Hospital of Basel, Spitalstrasse 21, Basel 4031, Switzerland; [b] Center for Advanced Orthopedic Studies, Beth Israel Deaconess Medical Center, Harvard Medical School, 330 Brookline Avenue, RN 115, Boston, MA 02215, USA
* Corresponding authors. Orthopaedic Department, University Hospital of Basel, Spitalstrasse 21, Basel 4031, Switzerland.
E-mail addresses: mwiewiorski@uhbs.ch; vvalderrabano@uhbs.ch

Foot Ankle Clin N Am 18 (2013) 543–554
http://dx.doi.org/10.1016/j.fcl.2013.06.009
1083-7515/13/$ – see front matter © 2013 Elsevier Inc. All rights reserved.

to the ankle joint has been confirmed by literature in recent years. Talar tilt in the malleolar mortise during ankle sprains and ankle fractures has been shown to induce cartilage damage and osteochondral fractures in ex vivo as well as in vivo studies.[5–7] The idea dates back to the anatomic investigations by Berndt and Harty[8] in 1959. In this frequently cited study, ankle joints of amputation specimens were exposed to inversion or eversion forces, dissected, and checked for trauma to the upper talar surface. Based on those experiments, a radiological classification was developed, which described a chain of consecutive morphologic changes induced by traumatic forces to the ankle joint. These changes ranged from compression of subchondral bone to occurrence and displacement of an osteochondral fragment. The original classification was later modified by Loomer and colleagues[9] and amended by an additional stage describing the presence of subchondral cysts. Flick and Gould[10] found reports of osteochondral lesions of the talar dome in more than 500 patients. They observed that 98% of lateral talar dome lesions and 70% of medial talar dome lesions were associated with trauma. The pathoetiology of frequently found cystic degeneration of the subchondral bone in OCLT are unknown. It has recently been theorized that, because of ultrahigh congruency of the ankle joint, the synovial fluid forces its way into small cracks in the subchondral bone, creating caverns in the spongiosa.[11] In contrast with cartilage, subchondral bone is richly innervated by nerves transmitting pain sensation,[12,13] therefore repetitive high fluid pressure in the subchondral bone could be an explanation for pain perceived by the patients (**Fig. 1**A and B).[14]

OCLT DIAGNOSTICS

Patients present with pain, swelling, and occasional locking of the joint. History frequently reveals past traumatic events to the ankle joint (sprains/fractures). Sport activities are reduced or halted. Clinical examination assessment should include assessment of hindfoot alignment and ankle joint stability. Because of its ubiquitous availability and cost-effectiveness, and its ability of assessing hindfoot alignment under loading conditions, planar radiography is regarded as the gold standard of radiological

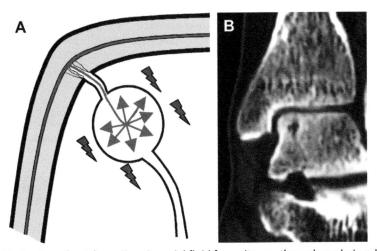

Fig. 1. Mechanism of cyst formation. Synovial fluid forces its way through cracks in subchondral bone and creates cystic caverns lined with pain receptors (A). The canal connecting the subchondral bone plate with the cyst and with the subtalar joint can be seen on computed tomography (CT) examinations (B).

OCLT diagnostics and is indicated as a primary imaging modality. Because of limited sensitivity for some stages and locations of OCLT and its planar, two-dimensional aspect, it should be complemented by modern imaging techniques such as computed tomography (CT) and/or magnetic resonance imaging (MRI). The defect volume and location can be precisely determined by CT, which allows planning for osseous reconstruction and intraoperative access to the defect (open vs arthroscopic).[15] Routine MRI sequences add information about cartilage morphology, soft tissue disorders, and activity of subchondral bone (bone marrow edema) and are sensitive during early stages of the disease. There is no evident superiority of CT compared with MRI or vice versa [16] and its use is subject to surgeon experience and approach. However, a disadvantage of CT is that the purely cartilaginous lesion cannot be detected.[16] Other available techniques (scintigraphy/single-photon emission computed tomography-CT,[14,17] ultrasound[18]) may add additional information, but do not play a role in routine OCLT diagnostics. Although several advanced classification systems describing the morphologic aspect of the lesion exist for CT/MRI, the most recognized gold standard classification is still the classification by Berndt and Harty[8] and Loomer and colleagues[9] for planar radiographs. A complete list of all currently used classification systems can be found in a recent review by O'Loughlin and colleagues.[19]

Ankle arthroscopy is useful in cases of unclear ankle pain and should be performed before any open procedure. Lesion location and extent of cartilage degeneration can easily be assessed and graded according to Outerbridge.[20] However, it is more difficult to assess the exact extent of the osseous lesion. An excellent correlation between arthroscopic and MRI detection of cartilage damage has been shown in several studies.[3,21]

SURGICAL TECHNIQUES AND GENERAL CONSIDERATIONS

Numerous surgical treatment methods are available and they can be categorized into non–tissue transplantation and tissue transplantation methods. An overview is given in **Tables 1** and **2**.

Table 1 Surgical technique overview	
Non–Tissue Transplantation	**Tissue Transplantation**
Refixation	Autologous tissue
Debridement plus bone marrow stimulation (microfracture/microdrilling)	• Autologous bone graft
• Matrix augmented	○ Anterograde
○ AMIC	○ Retrograde drilling
Synthetic scaffolds	• ACI
Metal implant	○ MACI
Percutaneous osteoplasty	• OATS
	○ One plug
	○ Mosaicplasty
	• Bone marrow concentrate
	• Isolated mesenchymal stem cells
	Allograft tissue
	• Allograft transplantation
	○ Bulk
	○ OATS
	○ Juvenile minced cartilage

Abbreviations: ACI, autologous chondrocyte implantation; AMIC, autologous matrix-induced chondrogenesis; MACI, matrix-associated ACI; OATS, osteochondral autograft transplantation.

Table 2 Recommendations for primary symptomatic OCLT, based on level 4 studies		
<1.5 cm^2	1.5 cm^2–3 cm^2	>3 cm^2
Debridement + bone marrow stimulation	ACI/MACI OATS AMIC	OATS AMIC Bulk allograft

Lesion size is an important parameter for outcome after OCLT repair, with 1.5 cm^2 cited by several investigators as a useful cutoff for determining prognosis and choosing among treatment options.[22,23] Other factors that have been shown to correlate with treatment outcome in OCLT include arthroscopic appearance,[24] the presence of associated lesions, whether the OCLT were contained within peripheral cartilage borders,[25] symptom duration,[19] and history of trauma.[26] Choi and colleagues[27] found age to have a negative effect on outcome, once confounding factors such as duration of symptoms and history of trauma had been taken into consideration. The choice of treatment should take into account whether a purely cartilaginous or an osteochondral lesion is present.

DEBRIDEMENT FOLLOWED BY BONE MARROW STIMULATION

The initial surgical treatment of most lesions involves arthroscopy with removal of unstable cartilage and the underlying necrotic/fibrotic bone (debridement/curettage/excision) and bone marrow stimulation (microfracturing/microdrilling). The goal of this procedure is to induce development of fibrocartilage at the defect site by disrupting the subchondral plate with subsequent release of growth factors and mesenchymal stem cells (MSCs) (Fig. 2A).

Although the long-term efficacy of microfracture in OCLT is controversial, many case series have shown that it provides symptomatic relief.[28–30] In a study investigating the influence of lesion size, Chuckpaiwong and colleagues[31,32] reported no failures after microfracturing with lesions smaller than 15 mm (n = 73) regardless of location, but only 1 successful outcome in lesions greater than 15 mm (n = 32; level 4 study).

This cartilage technique remains the gold standard of cartilage repair. Although other techniques show good results in case series, no high-quality study exists showing the advantage of another surgical technique compared with debridement followed by bone marrow stimulation. It is a cheap, readily available, 1-step technique.

AUTOLOGOUS BONE GRAFTING

Autologous cancellous bone is harvested from a suitable donor site (eg, iliac crest, proximal/distal tibia, calcaneus) and packed firmly into the defect generated by debridement and bone marrow stimulation of the OCLT (see Fig. 2B). This nonstructural graft is rich in growth factors and MSCs. Draper and Fallat[33] treated 14 patients with autologous spongiosa from the proximal tibia (level 4 study). After 71.5 months (standard deviation 21.1 months) they noted better overall clinical scores, better range of motion, and less pain compared with a group of 17 patients with debridement and subchondral drilling as the primary treatment technique. Kolker and colleagues[34] retrospectively reviewed a group of 13 patients treated with open bone grafting (level 4 study). Six patients (46%) were clinical failures requiring further surgery. Of the remaining 7, postoperative functional outcome results were obtained at a mean of

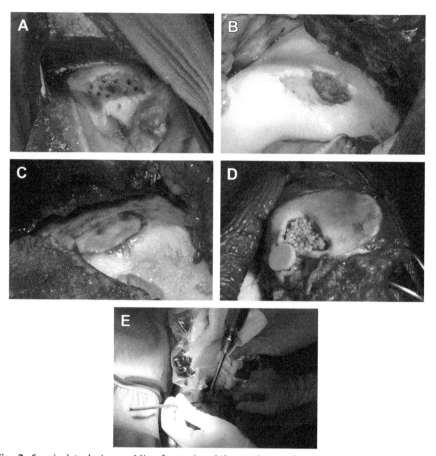

Fig. 2. Surgical techniques. Microfracturing (*A*); autologous bone grafting (*B*); AMIC (*C*); juvenile allograft cartilage, in this case on the patella combined with an acellular allograft cylinder (*D*); and retrograde drilling, in this case CT guided and robot assisted (*E*).

51.9 months with the American Orthopaedic Foot and Ankle Society (AOFAS) hindfoot scale improving from 55 to 84.3 after surgery. The investigators doubted the success of autologous bone grafting alone as the primary treatment, but they recommended bone grafting in combination with other cartilage restoring procedures.

One such procedure is autologous matrix-induced chondrogenesis (AMIC) (see **Fig. 2**C).[35,36] Following bone grafting, the defect is covered with a collagen I/III matrix of porcine origin. Valderrabano and colleagues[4] recently described their experience with 26 cases of OCLT with a mean size of 1.7 cm^3 (level 4 study). At mean follow-up of 31 months (range, 24–83 months) the patients showed an improved AOFAS hindfoot scale from 60 to 89 points and a decrease in visual analog scale (VAS) from 5 to 1.6 points. The use of bone graft in combination with autologous chondrocyte implantation (ACI)/matrix-associated ACI (MACI) was described.[37,38] Another way of bone grafting as a treatment of cystic lesions with intact cartilage covering is retrograde drilling (see **Fig. 2**E).[39] The cartilage is first inspected arthroscopically. If it is not delaminated or disrupted, a drill guide is inserted through one of the portals and a guidewire is advanced through the sinus tarsi in the cystic region under fluoroscopic control. The cystic material is drilled out and the remaining cavity is filled with cancellous bone. In the largest case series available, Taranow and colleagues performed retrograde drilling in 16 patients and found good results after 24 months (range, 19–38 months) with the AOFAS hindfoot scale increasing from 53.9 to 83.6 points.[40]

ACI/MACI

ACI is a 2-stage procedure. Cartilage is arthroscopically harvested from the knee or ankle joint. Approximately 2 million to 3 million cells can be enzymatically separated from the matrix of the biopsy and are cultured for 6 to 8 weeks, resulting in at least 12 million cells available for implantation. In the original technique (first-generation ACI), cultured chondrocytes are seeded on the damaged area underneath a periosteal patch. As an alternative, the periosteum can be replaced with a collagen matrix, which can be glued onto the defect instead of suturing.[41] In the most recent development of this technique, the chondrocytes are imbedded on the collagen matrix immediately after culturing (MACI; second-generation ACI). The longest available follow-up has recently been published by Anders and colleagues[37] (level 4 study). Twenty-two patients undergoing MACI were followed up for 63.5 months. The AOFAS hindfoot score and the VAS score remained significantly lower over the course of 5 years (95.3 and 0.9, respectively) than before surgery (70.1 and 5.7, respectively). In 2 cases a biopsy taken after 12 months showed hyalinelike repair cartilage.

One study suggests that decreased postoperative pain may be an advantage of ACI compared with other techniques. Gobbi and colleagues[29] compared surgical outcomes in 33 patients treated with chondroplasty (11 cases), microfracture (10 cases), and osteochondral autograft transplantation (OATS; 12 cases) (level 2 study). No significant difference was detected between the groups at 53 months follow-up (range, 24–119 months) regarding the AOFAS hindfoot scale.

Certain disadvantages of ACI/MACI remain, including high costs for culturing and the need for 2 surgical procedures.

OATS

One or more cartilage-bone cylinders are harvested from the low–weight-bearing area of the ipsilateral knee.[42,43] Multiple small cylindrical plugs of varying small diameters (2–4 mm) can be harvested to implant and cover a larger area (mosaicplasty) of the talus. The intervening spaces fill with fibrocartilage but hyaline-transplanted cartilage populates the bulk of the remainder. Advantages for the OATS or mosaicplasty technique include the use of autograft tissue with robust fixation, and being a single-stage procedure that can be performed open or arthroscopically depending on lesion location. Both techniques necessitate an orthogonal approach to the articular surface. Surgical exposure of the posterior talar dome; large defect size; and matching cartilage shape, curvature, and depth of resection are all technically demanding skills. Donor site morbidity at the knee joint has been reported.[44] Even perfect graft positioning may not completely restore normal contact mechanics, and small deviations from anatomic placement can result in more marked abnormalities.[45,46]

The longest follow-up for this procedure was published by Imhoff and colleagues.[47] Twenty-five patients (9 revision OATS) were followed up for 84 months (range, 53–124 months). The investigators found significant increases for the AOFAS score (50 to 78 points) and a significant decrease for the VAS (7.8 to 1.5 points) from before to after surgery (level 4 study).[47] Scranton and colleagues[48] retrospectively reviewed a cohort of 50 patients with previously failed OCLT repair (debridement, bone marrow stimulation, or bone grafting) presenting a large cystic lesion of greater than 8 mm in diameter. They showed a significant improvement in the clinical score (Karlsson-Peterson Ankle Score) after a mean follow-up of 36 months (range, 24–83 months). They recommended OATS as a salvage procedure in a revision situation with a large bony defect when the alternative is ankle fusion.

ALLOGRAFT TRANSPLANTATION

Bulk allograft transplantation is reserved for large-volume cystic OCLT (<3 cm³). An allograft talus is obtained and cut to shape to match the receiving defect according to intraoperative radiological and direct measurements. Whether the grafts should be fresh or fresh-frozen is debatable. Fresh osteochondral allografts might show more chondrocyte viability than fresh-frozen grafts and should be transplanted within 7 to 14 days of the death of the donor.[49,50] Other investigators report good results with frozen allografts.[51] The transplanted allograft is fixed with screws.

Raikin and colleagues[52] performed fresh-allograft transplantation in 15 patients with large OCLT (mean size 6 cm³) (level 4 study). At follow-up after 54 months (range, 26–88 months), the AOFAS hindfoot scale and VAS improved from a mean of 30 points to 83 points, and 8.5 to 3.3, respectively. Only 2 patients required a subsequent arthrodesis. El-Rashidy and colleagues[53] reviewed 38 cases treated with osteochondral allograft and an average OCLT size of 1.5 cm² (level 4 study). At 37.7 months (range, 6–72 months) the AOFAS hindfoot scale improved from 52.3 to 78.8 points. Three grafts failed. Only 2 of the 38 patients would have chosen not to undergo the procedure again because of persistent postoperative pain. Some of the drawbacks of allografts are high costs and limited availability.

NOVEL TECHNIQUES

A novel allograft transplantation technique involving the use of cartilage from juvenile donors (<13 years old) was recently developed (see **Fig. 2D**).[54] After debridement of the OCLT, the defect is filled with particulated cartilage mixed with fibrin glue to keep it in place. This technique can be used in open[55] or arthroscopic[56] procedures. So far only case reports are available.[54–57]

Van Bergen and colleagues[58] describe a procedure in which the gap of the debrided lesion is replaced by a metallic inlay resembling the articular talar surface. Early results at 1-year follow-up in 15 patients are promising, showing a significant decrease of pain.[59]

In a case report, Seo and colleagues[60] describe a technique similar to percutaneous vertebroplasty. A large-diameter needle is driven into the cystic subchondral lesion under arthroscopic and fluoroscopic guidance. The cysts are aspirated and then filled with a hydroxyapatite bone cement.

SUPPLEMENTAL PROCEDURES

Some investigators regard concomitant treatment of posttraumatic deformities (malalignment), ligamentous instabilities, and the reconstruction of bony defects as compulsory for successful OCLT repair.[4,61] Correcting malalignment and instability of the hindfoot to restore normal joint biomechanics might be essential for healing of the recently reconstructed OCLT. Remaining pathologic stress on the repair tissue could eventually lead to graft failure and recurrence of pain. However, the role of instability and malalignment in treatment of OCLT is not fully understood and evidence is sparse. Ligament repair for ankle joint instability accompanying OCLT repair has been mentioned in a few case series.[4,62,63] Regarding corrective osteotomies, Giannini and colleagues[63] reported a case of metatarsal osteotomy in the presence of a cavus foot. Valderrabano and colleagues[4] performed corrective calcaneal osteotomies to correct hindfoot valgus in 16 of their 26 reported OCLT cases undergoing AMIC repair. In cases of severe malalignment at the level of the ankle joint, a supramalleolar osteotomy (SMOT) can be considered.[64,65] In a recent comparison of CT studies before/after SMOT for partial ankle osteoarthritis, Egloff and colleagues showed a redistribution of subchondral bone density from the degenerated site of the talus to the opposite talar shoulder. This finding suggests that the talar shoulder can be successfully unloaded by this procedure (Egloff C, Valderrabano V. Mechanical Adaptation and Density Distribution of the Subchondral Bone Plate after Supramalleolar Osteotomy for Valgus Ankle Osteoarthritis. submitted for publication).

Platelet-rich plasma (PRP) has recently been described for treatment of OCLT.[66] The physiologic role that platelets play in healing has led to the concept that PRP may improve the biology of cartilage repair. Mei-Dan and colleagues[67] evaluated the use of PRP and hyaluronic acid injections as a first line of treatment of patients with primary and revision OCLT (level 2 study). They noticed a significant improvement in pain and function for both substances compared with the preoperative scores after 6 months, but no significant superiority of PRP compared with hyaluronic acid in terms of VAS pain improvement.[67] No clinical or radiological results have been reported regarding the outcomes after the use of PRP in conjunction with surgical articular cartilage reparative or restorative procedures.

SUMMARY

Several techniques show satisfactory clinical outcomes in case series; however, based on level of evidence criteria, there is no evidence of superiority of any surgical technique compared with debridement and bone marrow stimulation. The overall level of evidence in the literature is low. No randomized controlled studies exist, and recommendations for OCLT surgery can only be made on level 4 studies or expert consensus. Available studies are mostly retrospective in nature; include all OCLT sizes and morphologic types; have wide ranges of follow-up time points; mix primary surgeries with revision surgeries; and rarely note joint alignment, stability, and additional procedures. Commonly used outcome scales like the AOFAS hindfoot scale show clustering of results, poor responsiveness, and ceiling effects.[2] OCLT surgery is often performed because of loss of sports activity, which is not reflected in the AOFAS hindfoot scale. A multicenter randomized controlled trial would be useful.

ACKNOWLEDGMENTS

The authors thank Christie-joy Cunningham for her help in the correcting of this article.

REFERENCES

1. Kappis M. Weitere Beiträge zur traumatisch-mechanischen Entstehung der "spontanen" Knorpelablösungen (sogen. Osteochondritis dissecans). Deutsche Zeitschrift f Chirurgie 1922;171(1-2):13–29.
2. Ferkel RD, Van Dijk CN, Younger A. Osteochondral lesions of the talus: current treatment dilemmas. Instructional course lectures 2013; Unpublished paper presented at the American Association of Orthopaedic Surgeons annual meeting. Chicago; 2013.

3. Mintz DN, Tashjian GS, Connell DA, et al. Osteochondral lesions of the talus: a new magnetic resonance grading system with arthroscopic correlation. Arthroscopy 2003;19(4):353–9.
4. Valderrabano V, Miska M, Leumann A, et al. Reconstruction of osteochondral lesions of the talus with autologous spongiosa grafts and autologous matrix-induced chondrogenesis. Am J Sports Med 2013;41(3):519–27.
5. Alanen V, Taimela S, Kinnunen J, et al. Incidence and clinical significance of bone bruises after supination injury of the ankle. A double-blind, prospective study. J Bone Joint Surg Br 1998;80(3):513–5.
6. DiGiovanni BF, Fraga CJ, Cohen BE, et al. Associated injuries found in chronic lateral ankle instability. Foot Ankle Int 2000;21(10):809–15.
7. Hintermann B, Regazzoni P, Lampert C, et al. Arthroscopic findings in acute fractures of the ankle. J Bone Joint Surg Br 2000;82(3):345–51.
8. Berndt AL, Harty M. Transchondral fractures (osteochondritis dissecans) of the talus. J Bone Joint Surg Am 1959;41:988–1020.
9. Loomer R, Fisher C, Lloyd-Smith R, et al. Osteochondral lesions of the talus. Am J Sports Med 1993;21(1):13–9.
10. Flick AB, Gould N. Osteochondritis dissecans of the talus (transchondral fractures of the talus): review of the literature and new surgical approach for medial dome lesions. Foot Ankle 1985;5(4):165–85.
11. van Dijk CN, Reilingh ML, Zengerink M, et al. Osteochondral defects in the ankle: why painful? Knee Surg Sports Traumatol Arthrosc 2010;18(5):570–80.
12. Wojtys EM, Beaman DN, Glover RA, et al. Innervation of the human knee joint by substance-P fibers. Arthroscopy 1990;6(4):254–63.
13. Bjurholm A, Kreicbergs A, Brodin E, et al. Substance P- and CGRP-immunoreactive nerves in bone. Peptides 1988;9(1):165–71.
14. Wiewiorski M, Pagenstert G, Rasch H, et al. Pain in osteochondral lesions. Foot Ankle Spec 2011;4(2):92–9.
15. van Bergen CJ, Tuijthof GJ, Blankevoort L, et al. Computed tomography of the ankle in full plantar flexion: a reliable method for preoperative planning of arthroscopic access to osteochondral defects of the talus. Arthroscopy 2012;28(7):985–92.
16. Verhagen RA, Maas M, Dijkgraaf MG, et al. Prospective study on diagnostic strategies in osteochondral lesions of the talus. Is MRI superior to helical CT? J Bone Joint Surg Br 2005;87(1):41–6.
17. Leumann A, Valderrabano V, Plaass C, et al. A novel imaging method for osteochondral lesions of the talus–comparison of SPECT-CT with MRI. Am J Sports Med 2011;39(5):1095–101.
18. McCarthy CL, Wilson DJ, Coltman TP. Anterolateral ankle impingement: findings and diagnostic accuracy with ultrasound imaging. Skeletal Radiol 2008;37(3):209–16.
19. O'Loughlin PF, Heyworth BE, Kennedy JG. Current concepts in the diagnosis and treatment of osteochondral lesions of the ankle. Am J Sports Med 2010;38(2):392–404.
20. Outerbridge RE. The etiology of chondromalacia patellae. J Bone Joint Surg Br 1961;43:752–7.
21. Ferkel RD, Flannigan BD, Elkins BS. Magnetic resonance imaging of the foot and ankle: correlation of normal anatomy with pathologic conditions. Foot Ankle 1991;11(5):289–305.
22. Choi WJ, Park KK, Kim BS, et al. Osteochondral lesion of the talus: is there a critical defect size for poor outcome? Am J Sports Med 2009;37(10):1974–80.

23. Cuttica DJ, Smith WB, Hyer CF, et al. Osteochondral lesions of the talus: predictors of clinical outcome. Foot & ankle international / American Orthopaedic Foot and Ankle Society [and] Swiss Foot and Ankle Society 2011;32(11):1045–51.

24. Choi GW, Choi WJ, Youn HK, et al. Osteochondral lesions of the talus: are there any differences between osteochondral and chondral types? Am J Sports Med 2013;41(3):504–10.

25. Choi WJ, Choi GW, Kim JS, et al. Prognostic significance of the containment and location of osteochondral lesions of the talus: independent adverse outcomes associated with uncontained lesions of the talar shoulder. Am J Sports Med 2013;41(1):126–33.

26. Takao M, Ochi M, Uchio Y, et al. Osteochondral lesions of the talar dome associated with trauma. Arthroscopy 2003;19(10):1061–7.

27. Choi WJ, Kim BS, Lee JW. Osteochondral lesion of the talus: could age be an indication for arthroscopic treatment? Am J Sports Med 2012;40(2):419–24.

28. Becher C, Thermann H. Results of microfracture in the treatment of articular cartilage defects of the talus. Foot Ankle Int 2005;26(8):583–9.

29. Gobbi A, Francisco RA, Lubowitz JH, et al. Osteochondral lesions of the talus: randomized controlled trial comparing chondroplasty, microfracture, and osteochondral autograft transplantation. Arthroscopy 2006;22(10):1085–92.

30. Thermann H, Becher C. Microfracture technique for treatment of osteochondral and degenerative chondral lesions of the talus. 2-year results of a prospective study. Unfallchirurg 2004;107(1):27–32 [in German].

31. Chuckpaiwong B, Berkson EM, Theodore GH. Microfracture for osteochondral lesions of the ankle: outcome analysis and outcome predictors of 105 cases. Arthroscopy 2008;24(1):106–12.

32. Wright JG, Swiontkowski MF, Heckman JD. Introducing levels of evidence to the journal. J Bone Joint Surg Am 2003;85-A(1):1–3.

33. Draper SD, Fallat LM. Autogenous bone grafting for the treatment of talar dome lesions. J Foot Ankle Surg 2000;39(1):15–23.

34. Kolker D, Murray M, Wilson M. Osteochondral defects of the talus treated with autologous bone grafting. J Bone Joint Surg Br 2004;86(4):521–6.

35. Wiewiorski M, Leumann A, Buettner O, et al. Autologous matrix-induced chondrogenesis aided reconstruction of a large focal osteochondral lesion of the talus. Arch Orthop Trauma Surg 2011;131(3):293–6.

36. Wiewiorski M, Miska M, Nicolas G, et al. Revision of failed osteochondral autologous transplantation procedure for chronic talus osteochondral lesion with iliac crest graft and autologous matrix-induced chondrogenesis: a case report. Foot Ankle Spec 2012;5(2):115–20.

37. Anders S, Goetz J, Schubert T, et al. Treatment of deep articular talus lesions by matrix associated autologous chondrocyte implantation–results at five years. Int Orthop 2012;36(11):2279–85.

38. Giannini S, Battaglia M, Buda R, et al. Surgical treatment of osteochondral lesions of the talus by open-field autologous chondrocyte implantation: a 10-year follow-up clinical and magnetic resonance imaging T2-mapping evaluation. Am J Sports Med 2009;37(Suppl 1):112S–8S.

39. Lee CK, Mercurio C. Operative treatment of osteochondritis dissecans in situ by retrograde drilling and cancellous bone graft: a preliminary report. Clin Orthop Relat Res 1981;(158):126–9.

40. Taranow WS, Bisignani GA, Towers JD, et al. Retrograde drilling of osteochondral lesions of the medial talar dome. Foot & ankle international/American

Orthopaedic Foot and Ankle Society [and] Swiss Foot and Ankle Society 1999; 20(8):474–80.

41. Drobnic M, Radosavljevic D, Ravnik D, et al. Comparison of four techniques for the fixation of a collagen scaffold in the human cadaveric knee. Osteoarthritis Cartilage 2006;14(4):337–44.

42. Hangody L. The mosaicplasty technique for osteochondral lesions of the talus. Foot Ankle Clin 2003;8(2):259–73.

43. Hangody L, Kish G, Modis L, et al. Mosaicplasty for the treatment of osteochon-dritis dissecans of the talus: two to seven year results in 36 patients. Foot Ankle Int 2001;22(7):552–8.

44. Valderrabano V, Leumann A, Rasch H, et al. Knee-to-ankle mosaicplasty for the treatment of osteochondral lesions of the ankle joint. Am J Sports Med 2009; 37(Suppl 1):105S–11S.

45. Koh JL, Wirsing K, Lautenschlager E, et al. The effect of graft height mismatch on contact pressure following osteochondral grafting: a biomechanical study. Am J Sports Med 2004;32(2):317–20.

46. Latt LD, Glisson RR, Montijo HE, et al. Effect of graft height mismatch on contact pressures with osteochondral grafting of the talus. Am J Sports Med 2011; 39(12):2662–9.

47. Imhoff AB, Paul J, Ottinger B, et al. Osteochondral transplantation of the talus: long-term clinical and magnetic resonance imaging evaluation. Am J Sports Med 2011;39(7):1487–93.

48. Scranton PE Jr, Frey CC, Feder KS. Outcome of osteochondral autograft trans-plantation for type-V cystic osteochondral lesions of the talus. J Bone Joint Surg Br 2006;88(5):614–9.

49. Stevenson S, Li XQ, Martin B. The fate of cancellous and cortical bone after transplantation of fresh and frozen tissue-antigen-matched and mismatched osteochondral allografts in dogs. J Bone Joint Surg Am 1991;73(8):1143–56.

50. Williams SK, Amiel D, Ball ST, et al. Prolonged storage effects on the articular cartilage of fresh human osteochondral allografts. J Bone Joint Surg Am 2003;85(11):2111–20.

51. Raikin SM. Stage VI: massive osteochondral defects of the talus. Foot Ankle Clin 2004;9(4):737–44, vi.

52. Raikin SM. Fresh osteochondral allografts for large-volume cystic osteochondral defects of the talus. J Bone Joint Surg Am 2009;91(12):2818–26.

53. El-Rashidy H, Villacis D, Omar I, et al. Fresh osteochondral allograft for the treat-ment of cartilage defects of the talus: a retrospective review. J Bone Joint Surg Am 2011;93(17):1634–40.

54. Cerrato R. Particulated juvenile articular cartilage allograft transplantation for os-teochondral lesions of the talus. Foot Ankle Clin 2013;18(1):79–87.

55. Hatic SO 2nd, Berlet GC. Particulated juvenile articular cartilage graft (DeNovo NT Graft) for treatment of osteochondral lesions of the talus. Foot Ankle Spec 2010;3(6):361–4.

56. Giza E, Howell S. Allograft juvenile articular cartilage transplantation for treat-ment of talus osteochondral defects. Foot Ankle Spec 2013;6(2):141–4.

57. Kruse DL, Ng A, Paden M, et al. Arthroscopic De Novo NT(®) juvenile allograft cartilage implantation in the talus: a case presentation. J Foot Ankle Surg 2012; 51(2):218–21.

58. van Bergen CJ, Zengerink M, Blankevoort L, et al. Novel metallic implantation technique for osteochondral defects of the medial talar dome. A cadaver study. Acta Orthop 2010;81(4):495–502.

59. van Bergen CJA, Reilingh ML, van Dijk CN. Novel metal implantation technique for secondary osteochondral defects of the medial talar dome – one-year results of a prospective study. Fuß & Sprunggelenk 2012;10(2):130–7.

60. Seo SS, Park JY, Kim HJ, et al. Percutaneous osteoplasty for the treatment of a painful osteochondral lesion of the talus: a case report and literature review. Pain Physician 2012;15(5):E743–8.

61. Aurich M, Venbrocks RA, Fuhrmann RA. Autologous chondrocyte transplantation in the ankle joint. Rational or irrational? Orthopade 2008;37(3):188, 190–5. [in German].

62. Kono M, Takao M, Naito K, et al. Retrograde drilling for osteochondral lesions of the talar dome. Am J Sports Med 2006;34(9):1450–6.

63. Giannini S, Buda R, Faldini C, et al. Surgical treatment of osteochondral lesions of the talus in young active patients. J Bone Joint Surg Am 2005;87(Suppl 2): 28–41.

64. Pagenstert G, Leumann A, Hintermann B, et al. Sports and recreation activity of varus and valgus ankle osteoarthritis before and after realignment surgery. Foot Ankle Int 2008;29(10):985–93.

65. Pagenstert GI, Hintermann B, Barg A, et al. Realignment surgery as alternative treatment of varus and valgus ankle osteoarthritis. Clin Orthop Relat Res 2007; 462:156–68.

66. Smyth NA, Fansa AM, Murawski CD, et al. Platelet-rich plasma as a biological adjunct to the surgical treatment of osteochondral lesions of the talus. Tech Foot Ankle Surg 2012;11(1):18–25. http://dx.doi.org/10.1097/BTF.1090b1013 e3182463ca3182461.

67. Mei-Dan O, Carmont MR, Laver L, et al. Platelet-rich plasma or hyaluronate in the management of osteochondral lesions of the talus. Am J Sports Med 2012;40(3):534–41.

What Leads to Failure of Joint-preserving Surgery for Ankle Osteoarthritis?
When This Surgery Fails, What Next?

Norman Espinosa, MD

KEYWORDS

- Joint preserving • Surgery • Failure • Treatment • Strategies

KEY POINTS

- Joint-preserving surgery has evolved as a new strategy regarding treatment of end-stage osteoarthritis of the hindfoot and to postpone or avoid total ankle replacement or ankle fusion.
- When joint-preserving surgery fails, pain is the main symptom that directs the course of treatment.
- Failures are classified into surgery-related failure, natural history, and infection. Combinations of these failures can occur.
- Treatment modalities are selected based on whether the joint can be salvaged or not, and encompass complex reconstructions, total ankle replacement, and ankle fusion.
- Whenever possible fusion or total ankle replacement should be avoided.

INTRODUCTION

With the recognition of asymmetric osteoarthritis (OA) of the ankle and the detrimental effects of deformity on hindfoot kinetics and kinematics, joint-preserving surgeries have been introduced as an attempt to postpone either ankle fusion or total ankle replacement.[1–5]

Trauma is the main cause for development of hindfoot OA, including malleolar and pilon fractures that are followed by neglected or inadequately treated chronic ankle instability.[6,7] Deformities at the hindfoot, whether idiopathic or acquired (especially varus deformities) and even without radiographic signs of OA, may be seen as

Department of Orthopaedics, Balgrist Hospital, University of Zurich, Forchstrasse 340, Zurich 8008, Switzerland
E-mail address: norman.espinosa@balgrist.ch

Foot Ankle Clin N Am 18 (2013) 555–569
http://dx.doi.org/10.1016/j.fcl.2013.06.014

prearthritic conditions that could lead to local overload of the tibiotalar and subtalar joints, resulting in focal defects of the cartilaginous surfaces.

Chondrocytes of the ankle are resistant to degeneration and have the potential for easy repair once damaged.[8–12] Removing the overload of a certain joint area in terms of an unloading joint procedure that creates a favorable environment for cartilage repair could be of benefit and may delay and/or avoid the development of OA.

All types of surgeries that do not directly affect the joint (ie, that do not take place within or on the articular surface of the joint) can be defined as joint-preserving treatment modalities. Joint-preserving surgical techniques include arthroscopic debridement, ligament reconstructions, distraction arthroplasty, and hindfoot osteotomies. Under normal leg alignment and in young patients, distraction arthroplasty might be an option. The concept is that healing of arthritic cartilage can occur when the joint is unloaded and subjected to intermittent intra-articular fluid pressure changes. In cases of major deformity, it is difficult to apply distraction arthroplasty.[13–16] In addition, distraction arthroplasty needs specific external fixation for about 3 months, which is an issue that needs detailed explanation because it can be difficult for patients to tolerate. In cases of anterior impingement by a localized spur that result in soft tissue squeezing, arthroscopic debridement can help to improve symptoms. Local osteochondral lesions of the talus and tibia might be addressed successfully by means of arthroscopic debridement and microfracturing.[17] However, in the presence of global OA of the ankle joint, arthroscopic debridement does not yield satisfactory results. In the absence of bony deformity and the presence of chronic ankle instability, just the reconstruction of ligaments might be reasonable. However, according to Sugimoto and colleagues,[18] some varus deformity of the hindfoot is frequently present in patients with chronic ankle instability, indicating that a simple ligamentous reconstruction may not be enough to correct alignment and supporting the need for osteotomies.

Nevertheless, even with the most experienced clinicians, joint-preserving surgery has the potential to fail. There is a need for more evidence-based reports in the literature on failure after joint-preserving surgery of the ankle. However, this article focuses on evidence-based data and the author's experience of realignment surgery and its salvage once it has failed.

WHAT IS CONSIDERED A FAILURE?

Joint-preserving surgery is intended to redistribute the loads within a joint in order to unload the degenerated area while simultaneously achieving maximum pain relief. In addition, although not yet proved, biomechanics could theoretically be improved, enhancing function and delaying progression of degenerative processes. If any of those goals cannot be achieved, joint-preserving surgery may be seen as a failure. It is of worth distinguishing between failures that are the result of the natural disease of OA and those that occur because of incorrect planning of surgery.

Whatever the underlying reason for failure, the most frequent symptom, as reported by the patient, is pain. If after a joint-preserving surgery, pain persisting for more than 12 months could be seen as failure. Exceptions from this are obvious implant failures (eg, plate breakage, complete collapse of graft material). The time frame for when to consider a joint-preserving surgery as failed is difficult to define. According to Pagenstert and colleagues,[19] a 12-month interval is reasonable. Although they did not investigate resolution of pain after joint-preserving surgery, they were able to show that it takes almost a year until major improvement of pain occurs after implantation of a total ankle replacement. This observation, which has also been made by the author, indicates that reparative processes within the cartilage of the hindfoot joints occur slowly and need patience on the part of the patient as well as the treating physician.

TYPES OF FAILURE

There are many types of failure after joint-preserving surgery:

1. Surgery-related failures
   a. Wrong indication
   b. Overcorrection
   c. Undercorrection
   d. Malalignment
   e. Inadequate fixation
      i. Delayed union
      ii. Nonunion
2. Natural history
   a. Global OA of the joints
3. Infection

SOLUTIONS

Depending on the underlying cause of failure there are various strategies to solve the problem. The main question is whether arthritis has transformed from local to global.

Surgery-related Failures

Wrong indication

The indication for when to perform an osteotomy is crucial in order to achieve a successful result. For a varus-type OA, best results are obtained in the early stages of disease.[20,21] Proper range of motion as assessed preoperatively is also important when indicating an osteotomy.

Overcorrection

Overcorrection can result in impingement syndromes, impaired hindfoot function, and deformity, and thus can become a risk to accelerate degenerative changes within the joints (**Figs. 1–9**). In case of overcorrection after joint-preserving surgery, it is necessary to assess whether a major part of joint cartilage is still intact and, if so, how much. Magnetic resonance imaging or arthrography–computed tomography may help to estimate the amount of viable cartilage tissue.[22] More recently, single-photon emission computed tomography–computed tomography has been shown to be a useful tool to detect arthritic areas within the joints.[23–25] If there is viable cartilage left, then a redirecting correction in terms of an osteotomy has shown acceptable results and can be considered. In patients suffering from overcorrected congenital clubfeet who had ankle impingement, supramalleolar corrective osteotomy has been shown as an effective surgical procedure. Knupp and colleagues[26] showed that the correction was associated with a low risk of perioperative complications and led to significant reduction of pain, increased ankle motion, and improved clinical outcome. However, if the degenerative processes have advanced, other measures need to be taken into account. In a patient with good range of motion but global ankle OA, a total ankle replacement represents a valuable solution. In a patient with painful ankle OA but impaired range of motion, a fusion should be considered. The outcomes of ankle fusion are better when no adjacent joint arthritis is present at the time of indication. Otherwise it might be reasonable to implant a total ankle replacement while simultaneously performing a subtalar joint arthrodesis.

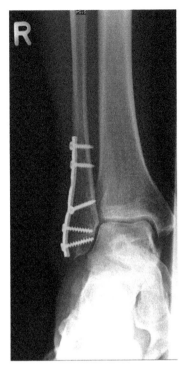

Fig. 1. Anteroposterior (AP) view of an ankle of a male patient who has undergone open reduction and internal fixation of his right fibula.

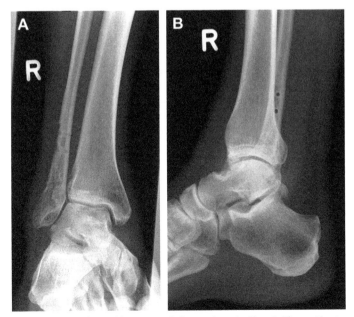

Fig. 2. AP (*A*) and lateral (*B*) ankle views of the patient in **Fig. 4**. The patient complained about irritation caused by the implant material. The implant material has been removed.

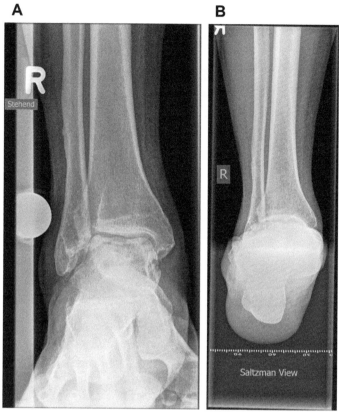

Fig. 3. Over time the patient reported pain in the lateral ankle region. AP (*A*) and Saltzman (*B*) views of the ankle joint reveal irregularities at the lateral talar dome and a subchondral sclerosis of the tibial plafond. In addition, the hindfoot is positioned in valgus.

Undercorrection

The same principles and results as apply for cases with overcorrection apply for under-corrections. Undercorrections are frequently a result of improper surgical planning.[27] By means of simple conventional radiographs it is possible to measure the angles: lateral distal tibial angle (normal, $89° \pm 3°$)/anterior distal tibia angle (normal, $80° \pm 3°$) and to estimate the amount of residual deformity. It is crucial to assess the apex of deformity because it represents the location where the correction is needed. When there is still good cartilage quality left, it might be possible to redo the joint-preserving surgery. Some patients may need an additive oblique or z-shaped calcaneal osteotomy (medializing or lateralizing) in order to correct varus or valgus malalignment. When there is already global arthritis and pain in the ankle joint, either total ankle replacement or ankle fusion must be considered.

Malalignment

Although any alignment in the coronal, sagittal, and transversal planes should be cor-rected, there are some cases with perfect alignment in the coronal plane but subtle malalignment in either the sagittal and transversal plane, or a combination thereof.

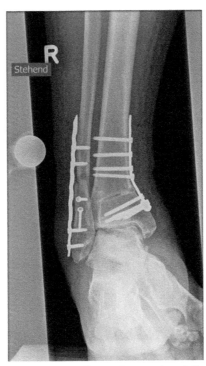

Fig. 4. In an attempt to correct the hindfoot valgus and to shift the loads from lateral to medial, a medial-closing wedge osteotomy combined with a fibular z-shaped lengthening procedure has been performed. Note that the gap on the medial side has not closed properly.

Any deformity in the sagittal plane can be assessed by means of the lateral tibiotalar surface angle (TLS), but rotatory malalignment in the transversal plane is difficult to detect. This condition is frequently found when accidentally cutting through the tibia, leaving an unstable situation. Under those circumstances it is helpful to use computed tomography of both legs and three-dimensional reconstructions in order to assess the angular deformity. Despite there being no scientific evidence to support the following statement, it is important to correct these residual deformities in order to improve function but also to halt degenerative processes at the ankle and to protect the knee joint function.

Inadequate fixation

Despite adequate treatment some osteotomies heal slowly or fail to heal. This inappropriate response to surgical treatment can be related to poor blood supply, the patient's age or nutritional status, and instability or motion at the osteosynthesis site. Other causes include nicotine, systemic hormones, certain medications, local necrosis, the form of bone, systemic bone diseases, and infection.[28]

Some investigators consider delayed union as a variation of normal healing. In a case of delayed union in an otherwise healthy patient, it could be advantageous to adapt loads at the osteotomy site and to increase weight bearing stepwise according to the radiographic appearance of bony healing.[29]

In contrast, nonunions are defined as nonunited bone fragments lasting at least 8 months after surgery. When there is formation of large callus tissue around the

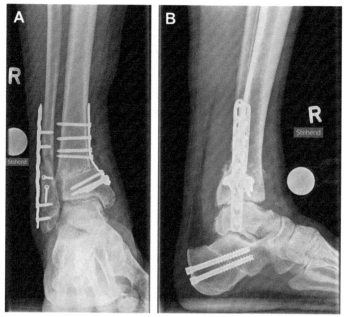

Fig. 5. The plate has broken. In addition, the patient developed a nonunion at the osteotomy site with medial shift of the distal fragment resulting in overcorrection. AP (*A*) and lateral (*B*) views of the ankle joint.

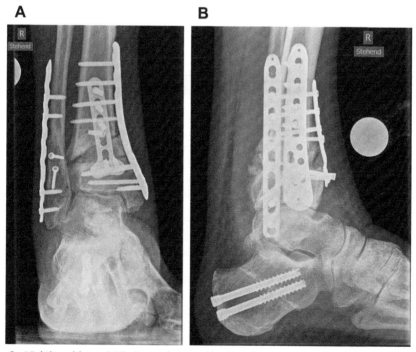

Fig. 6. AP (*A*) and lateral (*B*) views of the ankle. In order to correct the malalignment and nonunion, the nonunion site was debrided and cleaned out. An iliac crest autograft was harvested and inserted into the former nonunion area and fixed with 2 plates.

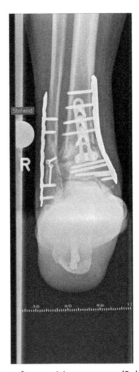

Fig. 7. A well-balanced hindfoot after revision surgery (Saltzman view).

osteotomy site it is called a hypertrophic nonunion. The reason for hypertrophic callus formation is instability at the osteotomy site. Proper treatment encompasses restabilization of the osteotomy, which can be achieved by hardware exchange or enforcing a current osteosynthesis. Sometimes decortication and application of autogenous cancellous bone graft can be helpful to stimulate bone healing. It is not recommended to remove the callus. The procedure is similar to that performed for tibial nonunions after fracture. Atrophic nonunions indicate biological failure of bone healing. In those cases, biology must be supported. Therefore, decortication and application of cancellous bone are mandatory. In addition, rigidity at the osteotomy site with a stable implant is needed (see **Figs. 1–9**). If there is any doubt regarding bony consolidation, the application of bone morphogenetic protein (BMP-2) has been effective in the treatment of tibial nonunions caused by osteoinduction.[30–34]

A special condition involves nonunion after insertion of a large bone graft. Allogeneic bone grafts serve as scaffolds and hence are osteoconductive only, whereas autologous bone grafts may provide some osteoinduction and osteogenesis.[35–39] There are difficulties in ascertaining whether a bone graft has healed in or not. However, the larger the graft the less likely it is to be incorporated quickly. The inserted bone graft is resorbed over time and substituted by the patient's bone, but this is a slow process. Therefore, the implant (bridging plate) prevents the bone graft from collapsing. In cases of implant loosening and bone graft collapse, revision consists of debridement, new bone graft application, and stronger osteosynthesis.[40]

In cases of nonunions it is appropriate first to try to solve the union problem rather than to convert the original osteotomy into fusion.

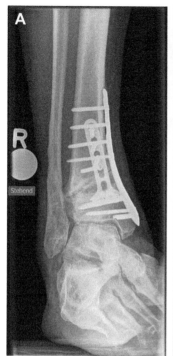
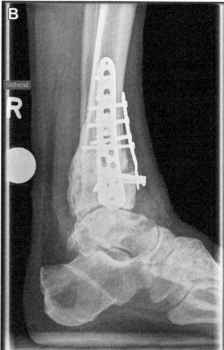

Fig. 8. The patient developed an infection close over the fibular plate. Thus, the plate has been removed followed by aggressive debridement and application of a negative-pressure wound dressing. The wound healed uneventfully and the patient was checked several times until definitive wound closure had taken place. The tibial osteotomy has continued to heal. AP (*A*) and lateral (*B*) views of the ankle joint.

Natural History: the Joint Advances Into Global Arthrosis

Surgeons strive to achieve a perfect result. However, even when accomplishing a perfect alignment of the hindfoot, OA can progress and become symptomatic. Symptomatic OA can be treated nonoperatively and surgically. Nonoperative treatment can be tried and consists of nonsteroidal medication, orthotics (to correct valgus or varus malalignment), brace applications (over-the-counter lace-up brace, custom Arizona brace, rigid ankle-foot orthosis [AFO], and floor-reaction AFO) and local injections. When nonoperative measures fail, surgery is warranted (Figs. **10–12**).[5]

Surgical treatment includes total ankle replacement and ankle fusion. It is beyond the scope of this article to discuss those treatments in details. However, it is important to consider correction of any residual deformity at the hindfoot because malalignment is not well tolerated by total ankle replacement and fusions.

Infection

Acute, superficial infections are early manifestations (<2 weeks) and include delayed wound healing, necrosis of wounds, and wound hematoma that become infected by an exogenous microorganism. Superficial infections, most frequently erysipelas (an acute streptococcal bacterial infection of the upper dermis and superficial lymphatics), can successfully be treated by either oral or intravenous antibiotics using penicillin, clindamycin, or erythromycin. The author prefers intravenous antibiotic

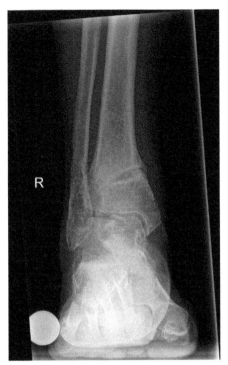

Fig. 9. The same patient as shown in **Figs. 1–8** became bothered by the remaining implants, which were completely removed. The patient now has global ankle arthritis and is scheduled for ankle fusion.

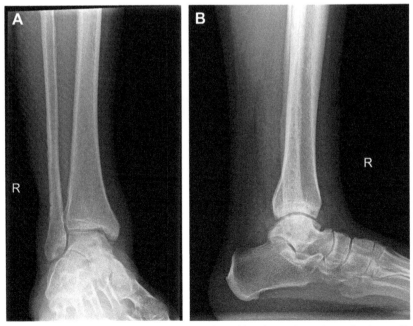

Fig. 10. AP (*A*) and lateral views (*B*) of the right ankle of a male patient who has suffered from posttraumatic ankle arthritis (ankle fracture type Wb B 10 years ago). The pain was localized at the medial part of the tibiotalar joint.

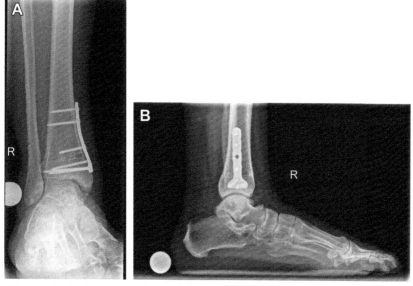

Fig. 11. In order to decompress the medial ankle joint, a medial opening-wedge osteotomy of the supramalleolar region has been done. AP (A) and lateral (B) views of the ankle joint 5 years after surgery. After an initial improvement for about 4 years, the condition became painful again and the images reveal global ankle arthritis.

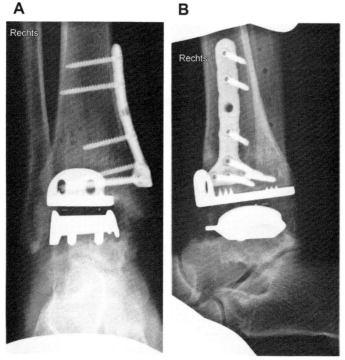

Fig. 12. The patient with global ankle arthritis but with good range of motion decided to get a total ankle replacement. The same patient as shown in **Figs. 10** and **11** (A, B) 1 year after surgery.

administration and a short hospitalization to properly control infection. Illness symptoms may resolve within 2 to 3 days, whereas the skin can take longer to return to normal.[41] In cases of wound necrosis, the local excision of necrotic parts and application of antiseptic bandages in combination with local skin grafts can help to solve the problem. When an infected hematoma is present, it is important to wash it out, to debride the wound area, to insert a suction drain, and to administer antibiotics (see **Figs. 1–9**).

In contrast, chronic and deep infections involving soft-tissues or bone, or a combination of both, need another approach. Orthopedic surgeons need to consider the involvement of a plastic and reconstructive surgeon in order to manage coverage of wounds and bridging of defects with vascularized grafts.[42]

Excision of the infected area is fundamental to surgical management.[43] As a first step, all infected and necrotic tissues need to be removed in order to leave healthy and well-vascularized tissue. If the underlying bone is affected, Judet and Judet[44] recommend aggressive and radical excision of all dead bone parts and osteosynthetic material. This excision is especially important when infections are assumed to be of inserted allografts or autografts. Specimens for microbiological typification of bacterial resistances, and thus proper antibiotic therapy, are collected. Local debridement is followed by a thorough irrigation, depending on defect size; negative-pressure wound therapy (vacuum assisted closure); and temporary stabilization (ie, unilateral external fixator or cast).[42,45,46] Local debridement and cleaning may be repeated until an uncontaminated wound is achieved. In a second step, reconstruction of the bone and soft-tissues can begin. It is important to perform local decortication where possible and to apply autogenous cortical and/or cancellous bone graft in order to enhance healing and to fill the defect. BMP-2 can be added to promote healing. Those steps are followed by stable fixation using a plate. If infection has reached the core of the bone (osteomyelitis) and when there is still the possibility that residual bacteria could be present, an intramedullary nail is not appropriate because it might promote infection into other bone areas. Masquelet recently described that, at the time of excision, an acrylic cement spacer could be used to bridge the defect and to save space for reconstruction.[47] The spacer should immediately be covered by local or free muscle flaps and remain in situ for 2 to 3 months. By so doing, it creates a foreign body membrane that is well vascularized and provides a perfect environment for consolidation of the autologous cancellous graft that is inserted at the second stage of treatment. When excessive debridement is necessary, the use of free vascularized bone grafts (eg, a free vascularized medial femoral condyle graft) can be discussed with the plastic surgeon.[48]

SUMMARY

This article discusses the lack of scientific evidence regarding treatment of failed joint-preserving surgery, the paucity of data in the literature, and the author's personal experience.

The concepts of treatment are various and most of them have been derived from well-known treatment modalities in trauma and orthopedic surgery.

The main question for the foot and ankle specialist is whether the joint can be salvaged even in the presence of failure. The definition of failure is difficult. Therefore pain reported by the patient is the main symptom that dictates the course of treatment.

Whenever possible the joint should be maintained. However, if pain is associated with global radiographic OA, total ankle replacement or fusions are the only means to solve the problem.

REFERENCES

1. Knupp M, Hintermann B. Treatment of asymmetric arthritis of the ankle joint with supramalleolar osteotomies. Foot Ankle Int 2012;33(3):250-2.
2. Knupp M, Stufkens SA, Bolliger L, et al. Classification and treatment of supramalleolar deformities. Foot Ankle Int 2011;32(11):1023-31.
3. Knupp M, Stufkens SA, van Bergen CJ, et al. Effect of supramalleolar varus and valgus deformities on the tibiotalar joint: a cadaveric study. Foot Ankle Int 2011; 32(6):609-15.
4. Pagenstert GI, Hintermann B, Barg A, et al. Realignment surgery as alternative treatment of varus and valgus ankle osteoarthritis. Clin Orthop Relat Res 2007; 462:156-68.
5. Martin RL, Stewart GW, Conti SF. Posttraumatic ankle arthritis: an update on conservative and surgical management. J Orthop Sports Phys Ther 2007;37(5): 253-9.
6. Horisberger M, Valderrabano V, Hintermann B. Posttraumatic ankle osteoarthritis after ankle-related fractures. J Orthop Trauma 2009;23(1):60-7.
7. Valderrabano V, Horisberger M, Russell I, et al. Etiology of ankle osteoarthritis. Clin Orthop Relat Res 2009;467(7):1800-6.
8. Aurich M, Eger W, Rolauffs B, et al. Ankle chondrocytes are more resistant to interleukin-1 than chondrocytes derived from the knee. Orthopade 2006;35(7): 784-90 [in German].
9. Aurich M, Anders J, Trommer T, et al. Histological and cell biological characterization of dissected cartilage fragments in human osteochondritis dissecans of the femoral condyle. Arch Orthop Trauma Surg 2006;126(9):606-14.
10. Aurich M, Squires GR, Reiner A, et al. Differential matrix degradation and turnover in early cartilage lesions of human knee and ankle joints. Arthritis Rheum 2005; 52(1):112-9.
11. Aurich M, Poole AR, Reiner A, et al. Matrix homeostasis in aging normal human ankle cartilage. Arthritis Rheum 2002;46(11):2903-10.
12. Kuettner KE, Cole AA. Cartilage degeneration in different human joints. Osteoarthritis Cartilage 2005;13(2):93-103.
13. Tanaka Y. The concept of ankle joint preserving surgery: why does supramalleolar osteotomy work and how to decide when to do an osteotomy or joint replacement. Foot Ankle Clin 2012;17(4):545-53.
14. Kluesner AJ, Wukich DK. Ankle arthrodiastasis. Clin Podiatr Med Surg 2009; 26(2):227-44.
15. Tellisi N, Fragomen AT, Kleinman D, et al. Joint preservation of the osteoarthritic ankle using distraction arthroplasty. Foot Ankle Int 2009;30(4):318-25.
16. Paley D, Lamm BM, Purohit RM, et al. Distraction arthroplasty of the ankle–how far can you stretch the indications? Foot Ankle Clin 2008;13(3):471-84, ix.
17. Niek van Dijk C. Anterior and posterior ankle impingement. Foot Ankle Clin 2006; 11(3):663-83.
18. Sugimoto K, Takakura Y, Okahashi K, et al. Chondral injuries of the ankle with recurrent lateral instability: an arthroscopic study. J Bone Joint Surg Am 2009; 91(1):99-106.
19. Pagenstert G, Horisberger M, Leumann AG, et al. Distinctive pain course during first year after total ankle arthroplasty: a prospective, observational study. Foot Ankle Int 2011;32(2):113-9.
20. Tanaka Y, Takakura Y, Hayashi K, et al. Low tibial osteotomy for varus-type osteoarthritis of the ankle. J Bone Joint Surg Br 2006;88(7):909-13.

21. Takakura Y, Tanaka Y, Kumai T, et al. Low tibial osteotomy for osteoarthritis of the ankle. Results of a new operation in 18 patients. J Bone Joint Surg Br 1995;77(1): 50–4.

22. Krause FG, Klammer G, Benneker LM, et al. Biochemical T2* MR quantification of ankle arthrosis in pes cavovarus. J Orthop Res 2010;28(12):1562–8.

23. Wiewiorski M, Pagenstert G, Rasch H, et al. Pain in osteochondral lesions. Foot Ankle Spec 2011;4(2):92–9.

24. Fischer DR, Maquieira GJ, Espinosa N, et al. Therapeutic impact of [(18)F]fluoride positron-emission tomography/computed tomography on patients with unclear foot pain. Skeletal Radiol 2010;39(10):987–97.

25. Pagenstert GI, Barg A, Leumann AG, et al. SPECT-CT imaging in degenerative joint disease of the foot and ankle. J Bone Joint Surg Br 2009;91(9):1191–6.

26. Knupp M, Barg A, Bolliger L, et al. Reconstructive surgery for overcorrected clubfoot in adults. J Bone Joint Surg Am 2012;94(15):e1101–7.

27. Paley D, Herzenberg JE, Tetsworth K, et al. Deformity planning for frontal and sagittal plane corrective osteotomies. Orthop Clin North Am 1994;25(3):425–65.

28. Schatzker J, Burgess RC, Glynn MK. The management of nonunions following high tibial osteotomies. Clin Orthop Relat Res 1985;(193):230–3.

29. Buckwalter J, Einhorn T, Marsh J, et al. Bone and joint healing. In: Buchholz HW, Heckman JD, Court-Brown CM, et al, editors. Rockwood and Green's: fractures in adults. Philadelphia: Lippincott Williams & Wilkins; 2010. p. 297–311.

30. Starman JS, Bosse MJ, Cates CA, et al. Recombinant human bone morphogenetic protein-2 use in the off-label treatment of nonunions and acute fractures: a retrospective review. J Trauma Acute Care Surg 2012;72(3):676–81.

31. Garrison KR, Shemilt I, Donell S, et al. Bone morphogenetic protein (BMP) for fracture healing in adults. Cochrane Database Syst Rev 2010;(6):CD006950.

32. Giannoudis PV, Kanakaris NK, Dimitriou R, et al. The synergistic effect of autograft and BMP-7 in the treatment of atrophic nonunions. Clin Orthop Relat Res 2009;467(12):3239–48.

33. Cook SD. Preclinical and clinical evaluation of osteogenic protein-1 (BMP-7) in bony sites. Orthopedics 1999;22(7):669–71.

34. Johnson EE, Urist MR, Finerman GA. Distal metaphyseal tibial nonunion. Deformity and bone loss treated by open reduction, internal fixation, and human bone morphogenetic protein (hBMP). Clin Orthop Relat Res 1990;(250): 234–40.

35. De Long WG Jr, Einhorn TA, Koval K, et al. Bone grafts and bone graft substitutes in orthopaedic trauma surgery. A critical analysis. J Bone Joint Surg Am 2007; 89(3):649–58.

36. Alter SA, Licovski L. Bone grafting for reconstructive osteotomies of the foot. J Foot Ankle Surg 1996;35(5):418–27.

37. Einhorn TA, Grelsamer R. The use of bone grafts for support and fixation in revision total hip arthroplasty. Bull Hosp Jt Dis Orthop Inst 1989;49(1):10–20.

38. Oloff LM, Jacobs AM. Fracture nonunion. Clin Podiatry 1985;2(2):379–406.

39. Einhorn TA, Lane JM, Burstein AH, et al. The healing of segmental bone defects induced by demineralized bone matrix. A radiographic and biomechanical study. J Bone Joint Surg Am 1984;66(2):274–9.

40. Judet R, Judet J. Bone compression in the treatment of pseudoarthroses and fresh fractures. Rev Chir Orthop Reparatrice Appar Mot 1956;42(6):911 [in French].

41. Hsu AR, Hsu JW. Topical review: skin infections in the foot and ankle patient. Foot Ankle Int 2012;33(7):612–9.

42. Hou Z, Irgit K, Strohecker KA, et al. Delayed flap reconstruction with vacuum-assisted closure management of the open IIIB tibial fracture. J Trauma 2011; 71(6):1705–8.

43. Jain AK, Sinha S. Infected nonunion of the long bones. Clin Orthop Relat Res 2005;(431):57–65.

44. Judet J, Judet R. Early infection in leg fractures. Rev Chir Orthop Reparatrice Appar Mot 1968;54(2):99–100 [in French].

45. Dedmond BT, Kortesis B, Punger K, et al. The use of negative-pressure wound therapy (NPWT) in the temporary treatment of soft-tissue injuries associated with high-energy open tibial shaft fractures. J Orthop Trauma 2007;21(1):11–7.

46. DeCarbo WT, Hyer CF. Negative-pressure wound therapy applied to high-risk surgical incisions. J Foot Ankle Surg 2010;49(3):299–300.

47. Karger C, Kishi T, Schneider L, et al. Treatment of posttraumatic bone defects by the induced membrane technique. Orthop Traumatol Surg Res 2012;98(1): 97–102.

48. Hertel R, Masquelet AC. The reverse flow medial knee osteoperiosteal flap for skeletal reconstruction of the leg. Description and anatomical basis. Surg Radiol Anat 1989;11(4):257–62.

Joint Denervation and Neuroma Surgery as Joint-Preserving Therapy for Ankle Pain

Andreas Gohritz, MD[a],*, A. Lee Dellon, MD, PhD[b,c],
Daniel Kalbermatten, MD, PhD[a], Ilario Fulco, MD[a],
Mathias Tremp, MD[a], Dirk J. Schaefer, MD, PhD[a]

KEYWORDS

- Ankle joint • Joint innervation • Joint denervation • Neuroma • Nerve transposition

KEY POINTS

- Partial joint denervation or neuroma surgery are joint-preserving approaches to treat chronic neurogenous pain around the ankle joint.
- Surgical interruption of neural pathways transmitting pain impulses from the joint to the brain is guided by nerve blocks using local anesthetics and the results from cadaveric studies identifying the skin and joint innervation of the ankle.
- Pain impulses from neuroma of the overlying skin territory can effectively be stopped by neuroma excision and nerve reconstruction or relocation into muscle, vein, or bone or nerve-to-nerve techniques. Clinical series in the literature prove that the positive results obtained for partial joint denervation and surgical neuroma therapy in the upper extremity also apply to lower-extremity joints (eg, the ankle and sinus tarsi).
- Based on a thorough examination and patient selection, a reliable and simple operation effectively alleviates symptoms and may prevent more invasive traditional surgical techniques.
- These techniques offer an ambulatory, minimally invasive, and rehabilitation-free approach for an increasing number of patients.

INTRODUCTION

Chronic pain around the ankle joint, above all caused by posttraumatic osteoarthritis of the ankle, is a severely handicapping problem to many patients. Treatment of painful lower-extremity joints traditionally focuses on musculoskeletal structures

Disclosure: The authors have no disclosures. There is no conflict of interest and no funding.
[a] Plastic, Reconstructive and Aesthetic Surgery, Hand Surgery, University Hospital, Spitalstrasse 21, Basel CH-4031, Switzerland; [b] Johns Hopkins University, Baltimore, MD, USA; [c] Dellon Institutes for Peripheral Nerve Surgery, The Exchange Building, 1122 Kenilworth Drive, Suite 18, Towson, MD 21204, USA
* Corresponding author.
E-mail address: andreas_gohritz@yahoo.com

Foot Ankle Clin N Am 18 (2013) 571–589
http://dx.doi.org/10.1016/j.fcl.2013.06.007
1083-7515/13/$ – see front matter © 2013 Elsevier Inc. All rights reserved.

and is initiated by radiological imaging and conservative measures, such as anti-inflammatory medications and injections (eg, steroids), altered activities, splinting, physical therapy, and, finally, pain management. If this fails, or structural disturbances (eg, osteoarthritis) are visible, surgical therapies usually follow. However, none of these strategies can claim to be the ideal solution. This applies to joint-preserving reconstruction, performed either open or arthroscopically, as well as joint fusion (arthrodesis), which may be unsuitable for patients of young age or with only mild degenerative changes. Long-term outcome of prosthetic joint replacement is still uncertain.[1–3]

The sinus tarsi relates to the bones of the anterolateral ankle and is not a true joint. Inversion sprains tear these ligaments that maintain the relationships of the talus, calcaneus, and cuboid bones forming this space. Pain is referred to as "outside of the ankle."[4,5] When conservative treatment for "sinus tarsi syndrome" fails and pain becomes recalcitrant, surgical options involve "evacuation" or "curettage" of the contents of the sinus tarsi, ankle arthroscopy, and subtalar fusion. Pain from dorsal cutaneous neuromas and ankle instability related to proprioceptive changes have been reported, suggesting sinus tarsi pain is of neural origin.[1,5]

Joint denervation or neuroma surgery may provide a valuable alternative treatment in selected patients with nerve-related problems around the ankle joint.

OBJECTIVE

This review article summarizes the indication, anatomic background, operative techniques, and clinical results of joint denervation or neuroma surgery, which, although rarely reported and used, may provide a valuable alternative treatment in selected patients with neurogenous problems around the ankle.

DENERVATION OF THE ANKLE JOINT/SINUS TARSI
Principles of Joint Denervation

Joint denervation is a surgical transection of afferent fibers transmitting pain to the brain that promises to preserve or improve joint function in painful osteoarthritis and prevent more destructive surgical procedures.[1]

History of Joint Denervation

Joint denervation is based on the demonstration that afferent nerves from the joints exist, although these nerves are mostly absent in standard anatomy texts. Following the meticulous description of the *The Articular Nerves of the Human Body* by the Munich anatomist Nikolaus Rüdinger (1832–1896) in 1857,[6] Camitz, in 1933, first cut the obturator nerve to treat hip osteoarthritis.[7] The idea to treat pain by neurectomy was transferred to other joints with varying success, including the ankle by Casagrande and colleagues[8] in 1951, the knee by Marcacci[9] in 1954, and the calcaneus and shoulder joint by Nyakas and Kiss in 1954 and 1955.[10,11] Nyakas also described ankle denervation in 1958 and introduced preoperative procaine nerve blocks to test the likelihood of successful neurotomy.[12] Albrecht Wilhelm complemented Rüdinger's studies on upper extremity innervation in 1958 and developed denervation of the wrist, finger joints, shoulder joint, and lateral epicondyle.[13–16] Initial pain relief was reported after more than 300 cases of "total wrist denervation" in 80% of cases, with persistent pain reduction after 10 years above 60%.[17] Dellon devised new approaches for partial palmar and dorsal wrist denervation[18–20] and tested the planned procedure preoperatively by local anesthetic block of specific peripheral joint nerves to reduce the need for multiple incisions and almost complete joint deafferentation. He established this partial denervation also in other anatomic regions. His approach included (1) anatomic dissection to identify joint innervation, (2) identification of effective local anesthetic injections, (3) demonstration that pain relief was possible by these blockades in patients refractory to traditional musculoskeletal approaches, (4) creation of surgical approaches to resect involved nerve(s), and (5) documentation of success with appropriate patient series.[1,21–23] With his coworkers, he described selective joint denervation to the knee, shoulder, sinus tarsi, temporomandibular joint, and medial and lateral humeral epicondyle.[24–32]

Indications

The goal of treating joint pain is pain reduction, stability improvement, and better joint function. Denervation is a modestly invasive and joint-preserving treatment useful in many patients with painful osteoarthritis. Contraindications include advanced joint destruction with completely destroyed cartilage, joint stiffness or instability (eg, by implant loosening), infection, synovialitis, or rheumatoid inflammation. Even chronic regional pain syndrome (CRPS) may not represent a contraindication if the pain is caused by stimuli from these injured joint and cutaneous afferents.[33] Failure is likely in patients with secondary gain motivation related to drug addiction, workers' compensation, or involvement with litigation. Advantages of denervation compared with more invasive surgical interventions, such as prosthetic joint replacement or arthrodesis, are numerous (**Box 1**).

Complications are rare, but may include infection (empyema) by inadvertent opening of the capsule; wound-healing problems, such as hematoma, seroma (increased in the lower extremities), or skin necrosis; scarring with risk of renewed nerve affection; limited loss of skin sensibility; progression of osteoarthritis; and renewed pain caused by endosteal and subchondral pain fibers.[1,22,34]

A potential criticism of lower-extremity joint denervation may be that it produces Charcot joints. However, although poorly appreciated by most physicians, the basis for proprioception is related to cutaneous afferents rather than joint afferents, whose purpose is to send messages to the cerebellum to warn acutely when the tension in the ligaments reaches a crucial level before disruption. A Charcot joint occurs in total joint

---

Box 1
Advantages of surgical joint denervation

1. Goal is to eliminate pain that is the primary cause of functional limitation.
2. Joint integrity is preserved.
3. Muscle function remains unaffected.
4. No implants/foreign materials are needed.
5. Postoperative immobilization is not necessary.
6. Operation is possible under local anesthesia.
7. Operation can be performed simultaneously with other operations.
8. The method is technically simple, inexpensive, and with low risk.
9. All alternatives remain possible for future (eg, arthrodesis or arthroplasty prosthesis).
10. The results can be reliably anticipated by preoperative test nerve blocks.

Modified from Cozzi B. Denervation of the wrist and hand joints. In: Tubiana R, editor. Surgery of the hand. Philadelphia: Saunders; 1993. p. 827–32.

denervation (eg, associated with syphilis and diabetes), but will not occur after partial joint denervation.[1,22,23]

Preoperative Preparation

Clinical examination
In the preoperative evaluation of the patient, the skin areas in the joint environment with numbness or tingling and pain that trigger points with a positive Hoffmann-Tinel sign are highlighted.

Local anesthetic nerve blocks
Preoperative blockade of pain fibers using local anesthetic allows the patient to anticipate the effectiveness of a planned neurotomy.[1,12] It can also distinguish if pain is caused by one or more nerves, which are blocked separately. Selective anesthesia of the respective pain-conducting nerve branch demonstrates the extent of denervation for each pathology (**Fig. 1**). The injection of the painful pressure points is always performed strictly extra-articularly. The patient is then requested to move and put weight on the joint, for example in the ankle by a forceful walk, preferably with stairs, and to report any change in the pain sensation while the anesthetic is effective. Reduction in pain of at least 4 points (or 50%) on the visual analogue scale (from 0 to 10) should be expected. If nerve blocks fail to significantly reduce or eliminate pain, we advise against denervation.[21,22]

Anatomic Background

Successful denervation is based on a thorough anatomic knowledge of the sensory innervation of the ankle joint and the sinus tarsi.

Innervation of the ankle
Rüdinger, in 1857, stated that the tibial, deep peroneal, and sural nerves innervated the ankle joint and also mentioned a branch running in the distal quarter of the lower leg dorsally to the interosseous membrane up to the region of the syndesmosis of the distal tibio-fibular joint (**Fig. 2**).[6] A century later, Nyakas and colleagues[11,12] still based their ankle joint denervation technique on the same nerves until von Lanz and Wachsmuth[35,36] recognized the saphenous nerve as additional sensory afference of the ankle joint. Mentzel and colleagues[2,3] demonstrated that all 5 major nerves of the lower leg (the tibial, superficial and deep peroneal nerve, saphenous, and sural) contribute to sensory innervation of the ankle. Great variety may exist and individual branches innervating the joint and certain rami for the ankle joint branch off from the main nerves quite proximally at the level of the beginning of

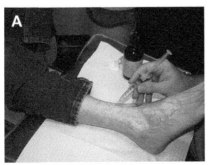 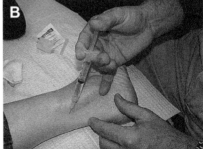

Fig. 1. Diagnostic local anesthetic nerve blocks in sinus tarsi syndrome: deep peroneal (A) and sural nerve (B).

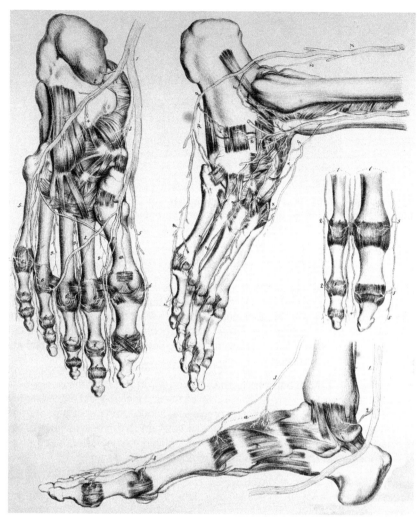

Fig. 2. Joint innervation of the ankle joint, as described by the Munich anatomist Nikolaus Rüdinger (1832–1896) involving the tibial, deep peroneal, and sural nerves and an interosseous branch.

the distal third of the lower leg. The interosseous branch is a terminal ramus of a muscular branch of the deep peroneal nerve.

Innervation of the sinus tarsi

Although innervation by the deep peroneal nerve had been suggested, a detailed description of the innervation of the sinus tarsi by the deep peroneal nerve was not reported until 2001, in the thorough anatomic dissection studies by Rab and colleagues,[37] which revealed that the sural nerve provides additional innervation in only about 20% (**Figs. 3** and **4**).[1,4,5]

Operative Techniques

Joint denervations are possible in local anesthesia, but often performed in general anesthesia, with the use of magnifying loupes and tourniquet.

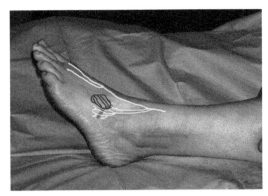

Fig. 3. Innervation of the sinus tarsi according to Rab and colleagues (2001)[37] and Dellon and Barrett (2005),[5] mainly by branches of the deep peroneal nerve.

Ankle denervation

This technique was described by Dellon and Mentzel and coworkers.[1–3]

Tibial nerve A longitudinal medio-dorsal incision is made in the lower leg starting about 10 cm cranially from the inner malleolus and following a curved path around it. The proximal segment of the tibial nerve is dissected and exposed beyond where it branches off into the medial and lateral plantar nerves and up to a point located distally to the apex of the inner malleolus. All side branches leaving the tibial nerve along this distance are severed.

Deep peroneal nerve A second longitudinal incision is performed on the ventral aspect of the lower leg extending from the same level as the first incision and extending to the dorsum of the foot. In the cranial section of this site, a longitudinal split is performed in the fascia of the lower leg, laterally to the anterior tibial tendon, over a distance of about 4 cm. The tibialis anterior muscle is secured and pulled medially, the deep peroneal nerve is exposed, severed, and a segment of about 2 cm is removed.

Interosseus branch (nervus interosseus cruris) The interosseus membrane is dissected upward and, if possible, the fine interosseus branch is severed.

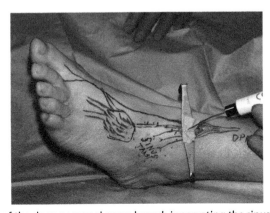

Fig. 4. Dissection of the deep peroneal nerve branch innervating the sinus tarsi before resection and intramuscular relocation.

Alternatively, the tissue is freed bluntly or with electrocautery over the whole width of the interosseous membrane.

Superficial peroneus nerve The superficial peroneal nerve is located in the subcutaneous tissue and is dissected up to the point of passage of its fascia in the proximal direction and beyond the ankle joint to the dorsum of the foot distally. The nerve mostly divides into 2 main branches, but can also consist of 2 or 3 tracts of equal size and is lifted up using a fine hook and all the branches are severed from the main trunk.

Saphenous nerve The saphenous nerve can be found via a separate 4-cm incision made longitudinally above the medial border of the tibia, where the medial third meets the distal third of the lower leg (slightly proximal to the 2 previous incisions). The nerve follows the vena saphena magna and may be split into several branches, so that the surrounding tissue has to be inspected thoroughly, even if a nerve has already been exposed, above all if the exposed nerve is very thin. The severance of the nerve(s) should be conducted as far proximally as possible so that neuromas may develop over the tibia but in the depth of the calf muscles where mechanical irritation is unlikely.

Sural nerve The sural nerve is resected using a longitudinal incision of 4 cm about 8 cm cranially and slightly dorsally from the apex of the lateral malleolus. The nerve is situated subcutaneously next to the vena saphena parva and is cut and removed as far proximally as possible, keeping in mind that in case of very distal junction of the 2 nerves forming the sural nerve, both need to be severed separately.

Surgical denervation of the sinus tarsi
This technique was described by Dellon and coworkers.[1,4,5] The preferred approach here is resecting the entire deep peroneal nerve proximal to the ankle, even if this may lead to loss of function of the extensor digitorum brevis muscle and sensation in the first dorsal web space. Preoperative evaluation frequently shows weakness of this muscle and impaired sensation in the respective skin territory already caused by stretch traction injury to the deep peroneal nerve. Attempts to preserve these functions have the risk of less than complete relief of sinus tarsi pain.

An incision is performed 10 to 12 cm proximal to the lateral malleolus. Both anterior and lateral fasciotomies should be used for easier access. There may be compression of the superficial peroneal nerve or a branch of this nerve might have been injured by a previous lateral ankle stabilization procedure, and the superficial peroneal nerve may need to be addressed simultaneously with sinus tarsi denervation. Dissection continues across the interosseous membrane to expose the tibia to reveal the neurovascular bundle by gently searching in the muscles here. After injecting local anesthetic, a 2.5-cm segment of the deep peroneal nerve is resected, preserving the peroneal artery and vein.

Clinical Results

Ankle denervation
Patient series reported in the literature after ankle joint denervation are summarized in **Table 1**. Results vary depending on the extent of denervation (ie, the number of nerve branches involved in surgical denervation).

Nyakas and colleagues,[10,12] in 1954 and 1958, published 2 series on the denervation of the calcaneus, ankle joint, and of the tarsal joints. First, they skeletonized only the tibial nerve and the deep peroneal nerve, whereas in the second article, they recommended also neurotomies of the deep peroneal nerve and the sural nerve proximal to the joint in combination with the skeletization of the tibial nerve. In the first series,

Table 1
Clinical results after ankle joint denervation

First Author, Year	Patient Number	Good Results (%)	Unsatisfying Results (%)
Nyakas & Kiss,[10] 1954	n = 48	73	27
Nyakas,[12] 1958	NS	100	0
Garrel et al,[38] 1972	n = 21	30	70
Mittlmeier et al,[39] 1992	n = 10	70	30
Mentzel et al,[3] 1999	n = 11	70	30
Richter,[40] 2007	n = 47	74	26

Abbreviation: NS, not specified.

complete pain relief was reported in 35 of 48 patients and decreased pain in the further 13 cases.

Garrel and colleagues[38] in 1972 published an article on the treatment of arthroses of the ankle joint by means of denervation, giving details of skeletizations. They used either 2 incisions, skeletizing the tibial and deep peroneal nerves, or 3 incisions, skeletizing the tibial, saphenous, deep peroneal, and sural nerves. Using this procedure, 7 good results were documented in 21 patients; 5 patients did not report for follow-up. Better results were achieved by Mentzel and colleagues[3] in 7 of 10 patients. In addition to the denervation, 1 patient had an osteophyte removed at the trochlea of the talus to improve the ankle joint's motion; the denervation was performed as the only procedure. This is where their procedure differs from the approach used by Mittlmeier and colleagues[39] in 1992, who presented 7 good results in 10 patients suffering from ankle osteoarthritis, following local repair surgery, together with the selective denervation of capsule-innervating branches of individual nerves as an additional measure. Mentzel and colleagues, and later Richter, attributed their better results to the inclusion of more nerves for denervation, which they concluded from their anatomic studies.[2,3,40]

Results of Sinus Tarsi Denervation

Dellon published a case report in 2002[4] and Dellon and Barrett[5] published a prospective clinical study to evaluate sinus tarsi denervation in 2005. In the series of 13 patients, 12 patients had recalcitrant pain after inversion ankle sprains or a fracture in the region of the sinus tarsi and 1 had an implant to correct severe hypermobile flatfoot deformity. Ten (77%) of those 13 patients were rendered pain-free after resection of the deep peroneal nerve. Two of the patients (15%), who were classified as having good results after having just the distal joint innervation fascicles resected, later required additional resection of the remaining fascicles of the deep peroneal nerve more proximally. Except for one, all patients demonstrated a short postoperative recuperation, with minimal pain and discomfort and a rapid return to regular activity, allowing immediate weight bearing, with 2 to 3 weeks before returning to full activity (this may be compared with the rehabilitation course for a subtalar fusion of 8–12 weeks of non–weight bearing and 6–8 months before return to full activity).[4,5]

NEUROMA SURGERY AROUND THE ANKLE
Principles of Neuroma Surgery

Besides nerve compression syndromes, severe nerve-related pain in the lower extremity mostly derives from neuroma, more exactly end neuromas, neuromas in continuity, and scar-tethered nerves.[41,42] End neuromas are unregulated and painful outgrowths of regenerating fascicles at the end of a severed nerve. Neuromas in continuity occur within an intact nerve in response to internally damaged fascicles and are similar in their symptomatology to scar-tethered nerves. In fact, those two may represent variants of the same problem, as the actual neuroma component of a large neuroma in continuity often appears relatively small once the surrounding scar tissue has been excised. Tethering of an injured nerve by scars may cause the nerve to fire spontaneously because it is inflamed or irritated, which may be triggered by chemical mediators of unknown nature. In addition, tethering of the nerve to adjacent structures results in distortion by shearing caused by movement of those parts (eg, joints), resulting in bursts of pain. Direct pressure may also increase the neuronal rate of firing due to direct compression or shearing effect.[41–43] Although most management strategies and clinical results have been focused on upper-extremity neuroma, successful treatment of in the lower extremity is of critical importance, especially as complete loss of tibial nerve protective sensation may envisage ulcer formation and possible amputation. Painful disturbance in gait, weight bearing, and overall lower-extremity function dramatically decreases the productivity and quality of life of the patient. Successful management of painful neuromas remains one of the most difficult problems in peripheral nerve reconstructive surgery.[41–43]

History of Neuroma Treatment

Ambroise Paré described neuroma in 1634, but recommended only massage and oil treatment instead of surgery. In 1811, Ollier confirmed that the bulbous stump of a severed nerve was especially sensitive and painful. The first histologic investigations were conducted by Wood in 1828, who introduced the term "neuroma." Improved understanding of the peripheral nerve anatomy and regeneration and the effects of surgery during the nineteenth and twentieth centuries led to a large number of methods to prevent and treat neuroma. Those ranged from transposition into unscarred noncontact areas, such as muscle, vein, fat, or bone, to sealing the nerve end with various materials, chemical or cryosurgical ablation, electrical cautery, or ligation. This great variety of methods, sometimes with contradictory results, suggests that no single one technique may be completely effective.[41]

Neuroma resection and transposition of the nerve end into a vein or muscle to change the microenvironment of the nerve and to minimize traction or mechanical irritation holds a preeminent role in modern neuroma management. This approach, using transfer into adjacent muscle, was described already in 1918, but established by Mackinnon and Dellon in 1985, while using a vein was already recommended in 1909 and this idea was popularized by Herbert and Filan in 1998.[44–47]

Indications

Surgical treatment of neuroma is usually started if conservative treatment, by medication, massage, and topical corticosteroids (to separate nerve from scar and to desensitize skin), for example, have been ineffective over 6 months.[1,22,43]

Risks and complications are rare, but may include infection and wound-healing problems, limited loss of skin sensibility, and renewed neuroma formation and pain. Individual factors, such as workers' compensation, employment status, litigation involvement, duration of pain, and number of previous operations, appear to predict the amount of pain after neuroma surgery. In a minority of patients with bad outcome, changes in the central nervous system in the spinal cord and the somatosensory cortex (central sensitization) and psychosocial factors may play a role in maintaining chronic pain.[48]

Preoperative Preparation

Clinical examination

Patient evaluation starts with a medical history and the anatomic identification of pain zone/trigger points, which indicates the respective injured nerve emitting painful impulses. Neuroma pain is usually characterized by

- Stinging, burning, lancinating, or electrifying sensations
- Limitation of complaints on innervation zone of a particular nerve
- Hypersensitivity in the area of previous incisions, trauma, or scarring
- Reproducible maximum pain on percussion of a trigger point with the pain radiating (Hoffmann-Tinel sign)
- Improvement of symptoms with proximal infiltration of suspected nerve with local anesthetic[1,21,33]

Local anesthetic nerve blocks

Diagnostic injection of local anesthesia is always performed proximally to ensure that blocking a specific nerve, not just a local pain point, may eliminate pain.

Anatomic Background

The surface anatomy of the lower leg (ie, the dermatomes of the sensory nerves) is the basis for identification and surgical management of neuroma around the ankle (**Table 2**).[1,41–43]

Table 2		
Nerves around the ankle, localization, and origin of injury and neuroma		
Affected Nerve	**Localization**	**Origin of Nerve Injury/Neuroma**
Tibial nerve	Lower leg or sole of foot (depending on level of nerve injury)	Trauma (eg, fractures, gunshot injuries, iatrogenic injury)
Plantar interdigital nerves (from tibial nerve)	Forefoot, usually between metatarsals	Neurectomy, instead of release in "Morton neuroma"
Calcaneal nerves (from tibial or plantar nerves)	Heel area	Excision of calcaneal spur, plantar fasciectomy, ankle fusion, calcaneus fracture
Deep peroneal nerve	Dorsum of foot, great toe	Orthopedic operations (eg, Lisfranc fracture/dislocation), foot operations (eg, hallux valgus, forefoot surgery)
Superficial peroneus nerve	Lower leg or lateral ankle (dependant on level of nerve injury)	Trauma operations (eg, foot ankle stabilization and open reduction internal fixation), knee trauma, fasciotomy, blunt trauma (eg, by suitcase)
Saphenous nerve (from femoral nerve)	Knee area or lower leg medially	Orthopedic knee operations, saphenous vein harvest for vascular or cardiac bypass grafts
Posterior branch of saphenous nerve	Medial ankle (proximal scar area)	Tarsal tunnel surgery
Sural nerve	Dorsal lower leg, dorsolateral aspect of foot	Sural nerve harvest for nerve grafting, biopsy

Operative Techniques

Reconstruction of critical nerves

In nerves with an important function (eg, the tibial or common peroneal nerve), the neuroma is excised and subsequent nerve reconstruction using either autologous nerve or conduit grafting is required. If the nerve is not critical, neuroma resection and a relocation procedure are usually performed.[41,43]

Relocation into muscle

Bulb excision and implantation of the nerve stump into well-vascularized muscle seems to be the most commonly used procedure in clinical practice. Clinical and experimental observations were reported in 1984 and 1985, suggesting that a classic neuroma will not form when a transected nerve is implanted into muscle.[1,22,44–46] Pain relief following intramuscular relocation may rely on reduced mechanical irritation, reduced scarring of the proximal nerve stump, and an increase in the distance from tissues producing high concentrations of free neurotrophic factors, such as the overlying denervated skin and the distal nerve stump.

Relocation into vein

The implantation of the nerve stump into a vein clinically and in animal studies demonstrated that the nerve stump grew into the lumen or wall, without forming a neuroma.[47] This method has shown to lead to a reduction in continuous, steady, and constant pain, most probably as the resection removes most axons vulnerable to stimulation and capable of producing spontaneous pain signals, which is regarded as the most debilitating feature for the patients. It has been suggested that the endothelium may play an inhibiting role on the formation of neuroma, and that the blood flow may remove neurotrophic factors released by the nerve stump. Coaptation can be performed end-to-side, as well as an end-to-end anastomosis if an end-to-side arrangement would require excessive mobilization.[43,47] Good clinical outcomes were reported by Koch and colleagues[49] and Balcin and colleagues,[50] who gained even better results compared with using nerve-to-muscle relocation.

Relocation into bone

Nerve-to-bone techniques are another alternative, with reported success rates of 70% and more (eg, for superficial peroneal neuromas translocated into the fibula), with better relief of symptoms than when transposed into the peroneus brevis muscle.[43]

Nerve-to-nerve techniques

Various nerve-to-nerve suture techniques have been reported, either end-to-end or end-to-side anastomosis with good outcomes, yet only in very small study groups.[51,52]

Centrocentralization was originally described to prevent amputation neuromas in the hand by coaptation of 2 nerve cords of central origin.[53] This technique can also be used for a single nerve if it is split into 2 fascicles of equal size, which are connected by simple end-to-end repair. One of the nerves or fascicles of central origin is then severed again in its proximal segment, producing a transplant of 5 to 10 mm so as to prevent the axons from both fascicles of nerves from meeting in the suture area. In the study by Gorkisch and colleagues,[54] only 1 of 30 patients developed a neuroma. Barberá and Albert-Pampló[55] confirmed good results after centrocentralization on painful neuromas in lower-extremity amputations, 21 of 22 patients were free of their neuroma pain at an average of 15 months of follow-up.

Aszmann and colleagues[54] reported on end-to-side neurorraphy into adjacent sensory and/or motor nerves to provide a target for axons deprived of their end organ to prevent neuroma and all but 1 of their 16 patients with upper- and lower-extremity neuroma improved in their symptoms at a follow-up of more than 2 years.

Clinical Results for Individual Nerves

Tibial nerve

The tibial nerve and its calcaneal, medial plantar, and lateral plantar branches provide sensation to the plantar surfaces of the heel, medial and lateral midfoot, and forefoot, respectively. Injury to the entire tibial nerve is rare, yet pain at the site of injury and sensory changes to critical contact surfaces may result. In neuroma due to tibial nerve injury, preservation or restoration of sensory protection is vital to prevent ulceration and possible amputation. The neuroma is excised and the tibial nerve is grafted, for example, by sural nerve from the contralateral lower leg. Preserving the sural nerve to the affected leg may provide limited, but valuable, protective sensation to the severely denervated foot.[41,42]

More frequently, injury to a tibial nerve branch may result in a limited deficit and clinical evaluation supported by electrodiagnostic tools, which can determine which sensory nerves are affected. Individual nerves can be successfully reconstructed also by sensory nerve autografts or bioabsorbable conduit, but care must be taken to prevent damage to uninjured nerves during the dissection. To preserve or restore either the medial or lateral plantar branches is imperative to prevent the negative sequelae of an insensitive planta pedis. Consequently, if a patient experiences neuroma-related pain in the foot arising from only one branch, this branch may be sacrificed without adverse outcome. Vernadakis and colleagues[41] recommend starting the dissection proximal to the injury, and carefully identifying the branches so as to neurolyze the affected branch away from the main trunk for at least 10 to 12 cm, transect and electrocauterize it, and transpose the distal end proximally in a tension-free manner into the soleus muscle.

Barker and colleagues[56] performed revision tarsal tunnel surgery on 44 patients, including neurolysis and decompression of the tibial nerve in the tarsal tunnel, the medial plantar, lateral plantar, and calcaneal nerves, in their respective tunnels. A painful tarsal tunnel scar or painful heel was treated, respectively, by resection of the distal saphenous nerve or a calcaneal nerve branch. Postoperative, immediate ambulation was permitted. Outcomes regarding patient satisfaction were 54% excellent and 24% good. It was concluded that resecting painful cutaneous nerves and neurolysis of all tibial nerve branches at the ankle offers hope for pain relief of pain and recovery of sensation for most patients after failed tarsal tunnel surgery.

Calcaneal nerves

Neuroma of calcaneal nerves is rare, but may arise after injury to branches from the tibial nerve, medial or lateral plantar nerve, or more than one of these nerves. Kim and Dellon[57] reviewed a series of 15 patients with heel pain caused by a neuroma of a calcaneal nerve due to previous plantar fasciotomy (n = 4), calcaneal spur removal (n = 2), ankle fusion (n = 2), or tarsal tunnel decompression (n = 7). The operative approach was through an extended tarsal tunnel incision to permit identification of all calcaneal nerves, resection, and implantation into the flexor hallucis longus muscle (**Figs. 5** and **6**). Excellent relief of pain occurred in 60%, and good relief in 33%. Awareness that heel pain may also result from injured calcaneal branches suggests that surgery for heel pain of neural origin should use a surgical approach that permits identification of all possible calcaneal branches.

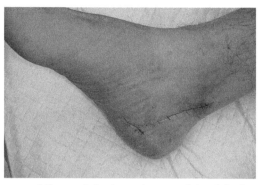

Fig. 5. Incision neuroma of the medial calcaneal nerve of the right foot.

Interdigital nerve (Morton) neuroma

Morton neuroma is a painful neuropathy resulting from compression of the plantar interdigital nerve between the metatarsal heads caused by the transverse metatarsal ligament. However, the almost universal approach for this metatarsalgia is to excise the (pseudo) neuroma through a dorsal incision. However, patients with unsuccessful neurectomy as the primary treatment of this condition often remain with a true neuroma and severe pain in the distribution of the affected nerve. This true neuroma requires a plantar approach over the noncontact surface of the foot well proximal to the neuroma. The plantar interdigital nerves are identified, divided, cauterized, and transferred proximally as far as possible into the dorsal midfoot in a tension-free manner to prevent displacement and to achieve optimal results.[41,42]

Considering that the mechanism of chronic repetitive compression of the common plantar digital nerve between the metatarsal heads, Wolfort and Dellon[58] explored the use of neurolysis in 5 patients with 11 involved nerves. The intermetatarsal ligament was divided, intrinsic fibrosis released, and the epineurium opened. Complete pain relief was achieved in 4 of the 5 patients, with the fifth patient, 13 years after a crush injury to the foot, achieving good pain relief. All 5 patients resumed their usual jobs and athletic activities.

Superficial peroneal nerve

The superficial peroneal nerve in the lower leg may be injured from trauma or iatrogenic procedures, such as during fasciotomies performed after orthopedic or vascular

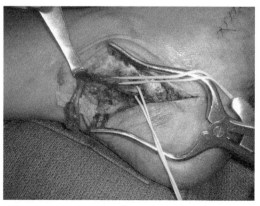

Fig. 6. Relocation of the neuroma into the flexor hallucis muscle.

surgical procedures. The nerve may also be injured at ankle level or at the dorsum of the foot from trauma or surgical intervention and subsequent neuroma may result in numbness and pain in the distribution of the nerve distally. Treatment of these neuromas in the calf consists of resection and transposition of the nerve into a muscle of the lateral compartment. Treatment is similar at the level of the ankle, except that the nerve is relocated into the midportion of the anterior muscle compartment. In addition, the anterior compartment may be decompressed by fasciotomy, thereby preventing recurrence of pain and creating a tension-free and pressure-free environment for the transposed nerve. Frequently, there are 2 branches of the superficial peroneal nerve, with one in a separate fibrous tunnel, which may be easily overlooked. Failure to address both of these branches may endanger a good result. Neuroma of the superficial peroneal nerve is rare, but occurs in sports trauma or fracture and dislocation, as the nerve comes under pressure between the underlying muscles and the overlying fascia. Although traditionally this nerve is depicted as being in the lateral compartment, it can be found in the anterior compartment in some patients. Dellon and Aszmann [59] retrospectively reviewed the location of the superficial peroneal nerve in 35 lower extremities in 31 patients with entrapment of the superficial peroneal nerve and found that the location of the superficial peroneal nerve was not different from the reported normal variation. However, the location of the superficial peroneal nerve in the anterior compartment in 47% of the patients in this series suggests that surgeons must explore the anterior and the lateral compartments in each patient with entrapment or neuroma of this specific nerve (**Fig. 7**).[60]

Deep peroneal nerve

Translocation away from mechanical irritation and into a muscle environment was used as treatment of dorsal foot pain of neuroma origin (**Fig. 8**). Identification of the deep (or superficial) peroneal nerves was achieved by anesthetic block, resection of the dorsal foot neuroma(s) and translocation of the nerves into the muscles of the anterolateral compartment yielded excellent results in 9 of the 11 patients with a mean follow-up of 29 months.[61]

Saphenous nerve with dorsal branch

The saphenous nerve travels together with the saphenous vein along the medial leg and may be damaged by tarsal tunnel release, with harvest of the saphenous vein

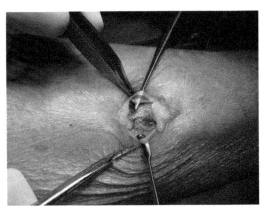

Fig. 7. High proximal separation of the superficial peroneal nerve into 2 branches, with one branch in both the anterior and lateral compartment, a potential cause of failure in case of partial ankle joint denervation or neuroma resection.

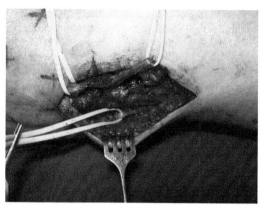

Fig. 8. Neuroma of the superficial peroneal nerve due to surgical incision before proximal resection and intramuscular transposition; note the close relationship to the sural nerve.

as cardiac or vascular bypass, or in orthopedic procedures around the knee. For proximal nerve injuries or injuries around the knee, preoperative nerve blocks above the injury level may predict operative success. For distal injuries in the region of the medial malleolus, there are frequently numerous contributory nerve branches. Treatment consists of identifying the nerve at a more proximal location above the medial malleolus and transposing the nerve more proximally. In cases in which this technique fails, the nerve may be identified above the Hunter canal and transposed into the muscles of the thigh.[41] After tarsal tunnel release, severe incisional complaints may be caused related to a neuroma that arises from injury to the crossing overlap branches of the saphenous nerves. An anesthetic nerve block relieves the incisional pain and the nerve is dissected proximally and transposed into a vein or muscles of the medial lower leg. Kim and Dellon[62] conducted a retrospective review of 16 patients with complaints after tarsal tunnel decompression, specifically the pain was located at the proximal aspect of the tarsal tunnel decompression scar. After positive test block, the pain was treated by resection of the distal saphenous nerve in the distal leg and implantation of the proximal end of this nerve into the soleus muscle, which achieved excellent relief of pain in 76% and good relief of pain in 24% of cases.

Sural nerve

Injury and subsequent neuroma of the sural nerve mostly occurs after nerve biopsies or graft harvest. Sural nerve injuries may also be caused secondary to lacerations or crush injuries of the heel or ankle or due to iatrogenic intervention (eg, during reconstruction of the lateral ligament of the ankle). In cases of a chronic, painful neuroma, the nerve can be transected proximal to the ankle to relocate the neuroma away from repetitive pressure on the posterior aspect of the calf into a muscular bed between the gastrocnemius or soleus muscles.[41,63] Alternatively, the nerve can also be transposed into a local vein in an end-to-end fashion, as suggested by Koch and colleagues,[49] which allows decreasing the size of the surgical incision.

Complex Regional Pain Syndrome

Dellon and colleagues[33] undertook a retrospective study to evaluate the hypothesis that CRPS type I (formerly reflex sympathetic dystrophy) may persist because of undiagnosed injured joint afferents, cutaneous neuromas, or nerve compressions; therefore, actually a misdiagnosed form of CRPS II (known as the "new" causalgia). Dellon and colleagues[33] described the long-term outcomes in 13 patients with a minimum of 24 months. Based primarily on preoperative physical examination and the response to peripheral nerve blocks, surgery included a combination of joint denervation, neuroma resection plus muscle implantation, and neurolysis. Outcomes measured in terms of decreased pain medication usage and recovery of function were rated excellent in 55%, good in 30%, and poor (failure) in 15% of the patients. It was concluded that many patients referred with a diagnosis of CRPS I may have continuing pain input from an injured joint or cutaneous afferents or chronic nerve compression, which is indistinguishable from CRPS II, and amenable to successful treatment by means of an appropriate peripheral nerve surgical strategy.

SUMMARY

Selective interruption of sensory nerve function can reduce or eliminate joint pain and improve function and quality of life. This concept is applicable for the peripheral nerve surgeon for painful joints or neuroma through the whole body. Pain impulses from afferents related to the ankle joint and neuroma of the overlying skin territory can effectively be stopped, which will help an increasing number of patients disabled by neurogenous pain in this area. The successful outcomes from the basic science and clinical surgery have to be transmitted to colleagues in orthopedics, podiatric surgery, neurosurgery, sports medicine, and pain management. Above all, in young patients with painful posttraumatic arthritis of the ankle joint, the option of a denervation should always be taken into consideration before performing a joint-destroying procedure, such as an arthrodesis or a prosthesis.

REFERENCES

1. Dellon AL. Partial joint denervation II: knee and ankle. Plast Reconstr Surg 2009; 123:208–17.
2. Mentzel M, Fleischmann W, Bauer G, et al. Ankle joint denervation. Part 1: anatomy—the sensory innervation of the ankle joint. Foot Ankle Surg 1999;5:15–20.
3. Mentzel M, Fleischmann W, Eifert B, et al. Ankle joint denervation: operative technique and results. Foot Ankle Surg 1999;5:21–7.
4. Dellon AL. Denervation of the sinus tarsi for chronic post-traumatic lateral ankle pain. Orthopedics 2002;25:849–51.
5. Dellon AL, Barrett S. Sinus tarsi denervation: clinical results. J Am Podiatr Med Assoc 2005;95:108–13.
6. Rüdinger N. Gelenknerven des menschlichen Körpers. Erlangen (Germany): Verlag, von Ferdinand Enke; 1857.
7. Camitz H. Die deformierende Hüftgelenksarthritis und speziell ihre Behandlung. Acta Orthop Scand 1933;1933(4):193–213.
8. Casagrande PA, Austin BP, Indeck W. Denervation of the ankle joint. J Bone Joint Surg Am 1951;33:723–30.
9. Maracci G. I Resultati a distanza delle denervazioni articolari. Minerva ortop 1954;5:309–12.
10. Nyakas A, Kiss T. Heilung von Beschwerden nach Calcaneusfrakturen mittels Denervation. Zentralbl Chir 1954;79:1273–7.
11. Nyakas A, Kiss T. Von Schultergelenkarthrose stammende Schmerzen—Heilung durch Denervation. Zentralbl Chir 1955;80:955–8.
12. Nyakas A. Unsere neueren Erfahrungen mit der Denervation des Knöchel- und tarsalen Gelenks. Zentralbl Chir 1958;83:2243–9.

13. Wilhelm A. Zur Innervation der Gelenke der oberen Extremität. Z Anat Entwicklungsgesch 1958;120:331–71.

14. Wilhelm A. Die Gelenkdenervation und ihre anatomischen Grundlagen. Ein neues Behandlungsprinzip in der Handchirurgie. (Hefte zur Unfallheilkunde, H 86). Berlin: Springer; 1966.

15. Wilhelm A. Tennis elbow: treatment of resistant cases by denervation. J Hand Surg Br 1996;21:523–33.

16. Wilhelm A. Denervation of the wrist. Tech Hand Up Extrem Surg 2001;3:14–8.

17. Buck-Gramcko D. Denervation of the wrist joint. J Hand Surg 1977;2A:54–61.

18. Dellon AL, Seif SS. Neuroma of the posterior interosseous nerve simulating a recurrent ganglion: case report and anatomical dissection relating the posterior interosseous nerve to the carpus and etiology of dorsal ganglion pain. J Hand Surg 1978;3:326–32.

19. Dellon AL, Mackinnon SE, Daneshvar A. Terminal branch of anterior interosseous nerve as source of wrist pain. J Hand Surg Br 1984;19:316–22.

20. Dellon AL. Partial dorsal wrist denervation: resection of distal posterior interosseous nerve. J Hand Surg Am 1985;10:527–33.

21. Dellon AL. Interruption of nerve function. In: Marsh J, editor. Current therapy in plastic and reconstructive surgery. St Louis (MO): Decker; 1989. p. 174–83.

22. Dellon AL. Partial joint denervation I: wrist, shoulder, and elbow. Plast Reconstr Surg 2009;123:197–207.

23. Dellon AL. Proprioception. In: Dellon AL, editor. Somatosensory testing and rehabilitation. Baltimore (MD): Dellon Institute for Peripheral Nerve Surgery; 2000. p. 32–6.

24. Dellon AL, Mont MA, Hungerford DS. Partial denervation for treatment of persistent neuroma pain after total knee arthroplasty. Clin Orthop Relat Res 1995;316: 145–50.

25. Dellon AL, Mont M, Mullik T, et al. Partial denervation for persistent neuroma pain around the knee. Clin Orthop Relat Res 1996;329:216–22.

26. Dellon AL, Mont MA, Hungerford DS. Partial denervation for the treatment of painful neuromas complicating total knee arthroplasty. In: Insall JN, Scott WN, editors. Surgery of the knee. Philadelphia: Saunders; 2000. p. 1772–86.

27. Aszmann OC, Dellon AL, Birely B, et al. Innervation of the human shoulder joint and its implications for surgery. Clin Orthop Relat Res 1996;330:202–7.

28. Dellon AL. Anterior shoulder denervation. Clin Exper Plast Surg 2004;36:175–80.

29. Davidson JA, Metzinger SE, Tufaro AP, et al. Innervation of the temporomandibular joint. J Craniofac Surg 2003;14:235–9.

30. Dellon AL, Maloney CT Jr. Denervation of the painful temporomandibular joint. J Craniofac Surg 2006;17:828–32.

31. Dellon AL, Ducic I, DeJesus RA. Innervation of the medial humeral epicondyle: implications for medial epicondylar pain. J Hand Surg 2006;31B:331–3.

32. Berry N, Russel R, Neumeister MW, et al. Epicondylectomy versus denervation or lateral epicondylitis. Hand 2011;6:174–8.

33. Dellon AL, Andonian E, Rosson GD. Lower extremity complex regional pain syndrome: long-term outcome after surgical treatment of peripheral pain generators. J Foot Ankle Surg 2010;49:33–6.

34. Gohritz A. Denervation bei Schmerzsyndromen der oberen und unteren Extremität. In: Vogt PM, editor. Praxis der Plastischen Chirurgie. Berlin: Springer; 2011. p. 411–7.

35. von Lanz T, Wachsmuth W. Praktische Anatomie, Bd. 1, Teil 4. Bein und Statik 2. 1st edition. Heidelberg, Göttingen (Germany); Berlin: Springer; 1959.

36. von Lanz T, Wachsmuth W. Pes - der Fuß. In: Lang J, Wachsmuth W, editors. Praktische Anatomie: Ein Lehr- und Hilfsbuch der anatomischen Grundlagen ärztlichen Handelns. Berlin: Springer; 1972.

37. Rab M, Ebmer J, Dellon AL. Innervation of the sinus tarsi: implications for treating anterolateral ankle pain. Ann Plast Surg 2001;47:500–4.

38. Garrel JF, Aubert M, Francois C, et al. Dénervation de la tibio-tarsienne dans les arthroses post-traumatiques. Rhumatologie 1972;24:337–40.

39. Mittlmeier T, Hertlein H, Beyer A, et al. Gelenkerhaltende Therapie der posttraumatischen Arthrose des oberen Sprunggelenks. In: Rahmanzadeh, Meißer, editors. Fortschritte in der Unfallchirurgie – 10. Steglitzer Unfalltagung. Berlin, Heidelberg (Germany): Springer; 1992. p. 347–53.

40. Richter M. Langzeitergebnisse der Gelenkdenervation bei posttraumatischer Sprunggelenksarthrose [Dissertation]. Ulm (Germany): Ulm University; 2007.

41. Vernadakis AJ, Koch H, Mackinnon SE. Management of neuroma. Clin Plast Surg 2003;30:247–68.

42. Elliott D, Sierakowski A. The surgical management of painful nerves of the upper limb: a unit perspective. J Hand Surg Eur Vol 2011;36:760–70.

43. Wagner E, Ortiz C. The painful neuroma and the use of conduits. Foot Ankle Clin 2011;16:295–304.

44. Mackinnon SE, Dellon AL, Hudson AR, et al. Alteration of neuroma formation by manipulation of neural microenvironment. Plast Reconstr Surg 1985;76: 345–52.

45. Dellon AL, Mackinnon SE. Treatment of the painful neuroma by neuroma resection and muscle implantation. Plast Reconstr Surg 1986;77:427–36.

46. Mackinnon SE, Dellon AL. Surgery of the peripheral nerve. New York: Thieme; 1988.

47. Herbert TJ, Filan SL. Vein implantation for painful cutaneous neuromas. A preliminary report. J Hand Surg 1998;23B:220–4.

48. Stovkis A, Coert JH, van Neck JW. Insufficient pain relief after surgical neuroma treatment: prognostic factors and central sensitisation. J Plast Reconstr Aesthet Surg 2010;63:1538–43.

49. Koch H, Hubmer M, Welkerling H, et al. The treatment of painful neuroma on the lower extremity by resection and nerve stump transplantation into a vein. Foot Ankle Int 2004;25:476–81.

50. Balcin H, Erba P, Wettstein R, et al. A comparative study of two methods of surgical treatment of painful neuroma. J Bone Joint Surg Br 2009;91:803–8.

51. Wu J, Chiu D. Painful neuromas: a review of treatment modalities. Ann Plast Surg 1999;43:661–7.

52. Gorkisch K, Boese-Landgraf J, Vaubel E. Treatment and prevention of amputation neuromas in hand surgery. Plast Reconstr Surg 1984;73:293–9.

53. Barberá J, Albert-Pampló R. Centrocentral anastomosis of the proximal nerve stump in the treatment of painful amputation neuromas of major nerves. J Neurosurg 1993;79:331–4.

54. Aszmann OC, Moser V, Frey M. Treatment of painful neuromas via end-to-side neurorrhaphy. Handchir Mikrochir Plast Chir 2010;42:225–32.

55. Lidor C, Hall R, Nunley J. Centrocentral anastomosis with autologous nerve graft treatment of foot and ankle neuromas. Foot Ankle Int 1996;17:85–8.

56. Barker AR, Rosson GD, Dellon AL. Outcome of neurolysis for failed tarsal tunnel surgery. J Reconstr Microsurg 2008;24:111–8.

57. Kim J, Dellon AL. Neuromas of the calcaneal nerves: diagnosis and treatment. Foot Ankle Int 2001;22:890–4.

58. Wolfort S, Dellon A. Treatment of recurrent neuroma of the interdigital nerve by implantation of the proximal nerve into muscle in the arch of the foot. J Foot Ankle Surg 2001;40:404–10.
59. Dellon AL, Aszmann OC. Treatment of dorsal foot neuromas by translocation of nerves into anterolateral compartment. Foot Ankle 1998;19:300–3.
60. Rosson GD, Dellon AL. Superficial peroneal nerve anatomic variability changes surgical technique. Clin Orthop Relat Res 2005;438:248–52.
61. Dellon AL. Deep peroneal nerve entrapment on the dorsum of the foot. Foot Ankle 1990;11:73–80.
62. Kim J, Dellon AL. Tarsal tunnel incisional pain due to neuroma of the posterior branch of saphenous nerve. J Am Podiatr Med Assoc 2001;91:109–13.
63. Coert JH, Dellon AL. Clinical implications of the surgical anatomy of the sural nerve. Plast Reconstr Surg 1994;94:850–5.

Index

Note: Page numbers of article titles are in **boldface** type.

Foot Ankle Clin N Am 18 (2013) 591–618
http://dx.doi.org/10.1016/S1083-7515(13)00068-5
1083-7515/13/$ – see front matter © 2013 Elsevier Inc. All rights reserved.

Moving?

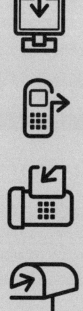
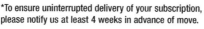

Printed and bound by CPI Group (UK) Ltd, Croydon, CR0 4YY

03/10/2024

01040493-0002